10-DAY *Green* SMOOTHIE CLEANSE

JJ Smith

10-DAY GREEN SMOOTHIE CLEANSE
by JJ Smith

Published by Adiva Publishing
12138 Central Ave, Ste. 391
Mitchellville, MD 20721

For more information, see www.JJSmithOnline.com.

DISCLAIMER: The author does not guarantee that any products or recommendations will provide you with the same benefits that she has achieved. You should seek a doctor and do your own research to determine if any of the products or recommendations made in this book by the author would work for you. Additionally, the author is not paid for recommending any books or products in this book.

While the author has made every effort to provide accurate product names and contact information, such as Internet addresses, at the time of publication, neither the publisher nor the author assumes responsibility for errors or changes that occur after publication. Additionally, the author does not have any control over products or websites associated with those products listed in this book or the content of those websites.

The book is sold with the understanding that neither the author nor publisher, Adiva Publishing, is engaged in rendering any legal, accounting, financial, medical, or other professional advice. If financial, legal, or medical expertise is required, the services of a competent professional should be sought, as no one at Adiva Publishing is a medical practitioner. The author and publisher shall have neither liability nor responsibility to any person, company, or entity with respect to any loss or damage caused directly or indirectly by the concepts, ideas, products, information, or suggestions presented in this book. By reading this book, you agree to be bound to the statements above.

Library of Congress Cataloging-in-Publication Data

Smith, JJ

10-Day Green Smoothie Cleanse/JJ Smith, First Edition

1. Health/Diet 2. Weight Loss 3. Women's Health and Wellness

ISBN: 978-0-9823018-2-1

Contents

APPENDIX A

APPENDIX B

Important Note to Readers

The information contained in this book is for your education. It is not intended to diagnose, treat, or cure any medical condition or dispense medical advice. If you decide to follow the plan, you should seek the advice and counsel of a licensed health professional and then use your own judgment.

It is important to obtain proper medical advice before you make any decisions about nutrition, diet, supplements, or other health-related issues discussed in this book. Neither the author nor the publisher is qualified to provide medical, financial, or psychological advice or services. The reader should consult an appropriate healthcare professional before heeding any of the advice given in this book.

INTRODUCTION

Welcome to the
10-Day Green Smoothie Cleanse!

Congratulations on taking control of your health by caring for your body and feeding it what it needs to be slim, healthy, and vibrant! If you're like me, you really want to look and feel great!

Battling excess weight can be one of the most frustrating, challenging, and emotionally draining experiences on earth. Many people struggle with a never-ending battle to lose weight and get healthy. Despite the numerous fad diets, exercise regimens, and magic pills for weight loss, Americans continue to grow larger and larger year after year. Diets abound, and the diet industry is huge. But the sad fact is that about 95 percent of people who lose weight on a diet gain it back in three to five years. You cannot lose weight permanently by strictly following any special diet, taking a weight-loss pill, or following an exercise regimen. You have to realize that losing weight involves a major lifestyle change.

What do I mean by lifestyle change? First, you will have to forget about dieting! Typically, you "go on" a diet, which implies that at some point you "go off" it. A typical diet is something you do for a specified period of time. What usually happens when you "go off" the diet? You gain all the weight back. With this ten-day cleanse, we are going to retrain your taste buds to desire and crave healthier foods so you never have to think about dieting again.

I believe the first step in losing weight is detoxification. Without detoxification, millions of people worldwide lose the fight to lose weight permanently. There are many factors that contribute to weight gain, and one factor that is most overlooked by traditional diets is toxic overload. Simply put, people often have difficulty losing weight because their bodies are full of poisons. The more toxins you take in or are exposed to every day, the more toxins you store in fat cells in the body. Toxins stored in fat cells are difficult to get rid of through dieting alone. You must first detoxify the body. Thus, the most effective weight-loss programs should focus on both fat loss and detoxification, which lead to overall improved health and wellness.

I am a nutritionist, a certified weight-loss expert, author of the #1 bestseller *Lose Weight Without Dieting or Working Out*, and creator of the Detox-Eat-Move (DEM) System. For years, I've helped people lose weight without dieting so they can get their sexy back! The DEM System focuses on helping you detoxify, cleanse, and reset your taste buds so that you desire healthy, natural foods.

Why I Created the 10-Day Green Smoothie Cleanse

Last year, after years of clean, healthy eating and detoxing, I was bedridden with mercury poisoning from my silver dental fillings! I had high levels of mercury in my brain, gut, liver, and kidneys. I couldn't get out of bed for two months. And when I did, just making the bed required that I lie back down to rest! My health, energy and motivation were at an all-time low.

After a long and slow recovery last year, I decided I needed to do something to get my health and energy back, as well as lose the twenty pounds I had gained while bedridden. I created the 10-Day Green Smoothie Cleanse after learning how raw greens can heal the body. Also, already an advocate of detoxing, I knew I needed to rid my body of excess waste and toxins that had accumulated as a result of the mercury poisoning.

Once I created the 10-Day Green Smoothie Cleanse, I asked if I could get ten of my family members and friends to do it with me for support. I was pleasantly surprised to find that about 100 of them wanted to do it! We created a Facebook group to keep one another motivated. Because the results were so phenomenal, in less than two months we had about 10,000 people join the Facebook group and decide to do the cleanse with us. In just ten days, folks were losing ten to fifteen pounds, getting energized, reversing health conditions, and feeling better than they had in years.

When I completed my first cleanse, I lost eleven pounds. My energy was high, my skin was radiant, and my digestion and bloating had improved. I felt renewed and motivated again! Before I began the cleanse, I had been taking twenty-four supplements a day to help my body recover from mercury poisoning. Since completing the cleanse, I have been taking only four supplements per day. I have such a positive outlook on my health and look forward to getting back to focusing on my life dreams and goals.

The 10-Day Green Smoothie Cleanse is a detox program that will help you lose weight, increase energy, reduce cravings, and improve overall health. You will detoxify your body through elimination of certain foods for ten days and reprogram your taste buds to desire healthy, nutrient-rich foods. After you complete the cleanse, you will never have to count calories or follow complicated or expensive meal plans or measure food again. Your body will naturally crave and desire healthy, natural foods.

During the 10-Day Green Smoothie Cleanse, you will give your body the quality nutrition it needs while cleansing your cells and insides. Vitamins, minerals, and other nutrients will be absorbed by your body more efficiently, allowing your cells to become like new as you begin to look and feel younger. What makes us feel old is sludge and waste in the body. Anti-aging creams and cosmetic surgery won't clean that out. Your skin will look more youthful because your cells will become tighter and healthier. Aging, dull, dry skin; puffiness; dark circles; and wrinkles will start to fade away. It is possible to look and feel better now than you did a decade ago. You will feel like you're growing younger, not older! In short, you'll learn how to become young, healthy, and energetic from the inside out.

I guess you could say that I have fallen in love with green smoothies and want the world to know it! Every day, green smoothies change the lives of so many people, including my own family and friends. I've had thousands personally thank me for introducing them to green smoothies. Anyone who has tried green smoothies can't help but share the experience with others.

I am committed to drinking green smoothies every day and getting as many people as I can to drink them as well. Will you join me in this journey to heal the body, lose weight and increase energy levels? By doing this, you will never have to worry about weight again.

Are you ready to look slimmer, healthier, and sexier than you have in years?

This is an amazing way to transform your health in just ten days. So get ready to start your 10-Day Green Smoothie Cleanse!

CHAPTER ONE

What Is the 10-Day
Green Smoothie Cleanse?

*T*he Green Smoothie Cleanse is a ten-day detox/cleanse made up of green leafy veggies, fruit, and water. Green smoothies are filling and healthy, and you will enjoy drinking them. Your body will also thank you for drinking them. You can expect to lose some weight, increase your energy levels, reduce your cravings, clear your mind, and improve your digestion and overall health. It is an experience that will change your life if you stick with it!

Most common health improvements after the 10-Day Green Smoothie Cleanse:

- Weight loss (most lose 10–15 pounds when they stick to the regimen)
- Increased energy
- Mental clarity
- Better sleep
- Reduced cravings
- Better digestion
- Less bloating

Why Detox/Cleanse the Body?

There are many factors that contribute to weight gain, and the one that is most overlooked is excess toxins in the body. When the body is overloaded with toxins, it transfers energy away from burning calories to work harder to detoxify the body. In other words, the body does not have the energy to burn calories. However, when the body is efficiently getting rid of toxins, the energy can be used to burn fat.

Simply put, traditional diets so often don't work because they don't address the toxic waste in the body. Counting calories does not detoxify and cleanse the body. Weight loss won't be permanent if your body's systems are sluggish or impacted with waste matter or toxins. You must first rid your body of toxins to ensure that your body can best metabolize the food you eat without leaving excess waste, which results in weight gain.

The following symptoms indicate the presence of excess toxins in the body: bloating, constipation, indigestion, low energy, fatigue/brain fog, depression, weight gain, chronic pain, infections, allergies, headaches, and gut/digestion problems.

Do You Need to Detox/Cleanse?
Take this Self-Assessment Quiz!

Take this quiz to determine whether you have toxic overload in your body leading to weight gain and poor health.

Read each question and give yourself one point for every "yes" answer.

- Do you crave sweets, bread, pasta, white rice, and/or potatoes?
- Do you eat processed foods (TV dinners, lunchmeats, bacon, canned soup, snack bars) or fast foods at least three times a week?
- Do you drink caffeinated beverages like coffee and tea more than twice daily?
- Do you drink diet sodas or use artificial sweeteners at least once a day?
- Do you sleep less than eight hours per day?
- Do you drink less than 64 ounces of good, clean water daily?
- Are you very sensitive to smoke, chemicals, or fumes in the environment?
- Have you ever taken antibiotics, antidepressants, or other medications?
- Have you ever taken birth control pills or other estrogens, such as hormone replacement therapy?
- Do you have frequent yeast infections?
- Do you have "silver" dental fillings?

- [ ] Do you use commercial household cleaners, cosmetics, or deodorants?
- [ ] Do you eat non-organic vegetables, fruits, or meat?
- [ ] Have you ever smoked or been exposed to secondhand smoke?
- [ ] Are you overweight or do you have cellulite fat deposits?
- [ ] Does your occupation expose you to environmental toxins?
- [ ] Do you live in a major metropolitan area or near a big airport?
- [ ] Do you feel tired, fatigued, or sluggish throughout the day?
- [ ] Do you have difficulty concentrating or focusing?
- [ ] Do you suffer bloating, indigestion, or frequent gas after eating?
- [ ] Do you get more than two colds or the flu per year?
- [ ] Do you have reoccurring congestion, sinus issues, or postnasal drip?
- [ ] Do you sometimes notice you have bad breath, a coated tongue, or strong-smelling urine?
- [ ] Do you have puffy eyes or dark circles under your eyes?
- [ ] Are you often sad or depressed?
- [ ] Do you often feel anxious, antsy, or stressed?

Do you have acne, breakouts, rashes, or hives?

Do you have less than one bowel movement per day and/or get constipated occasionally?

Do you have insomnia or trouble getting restful sleep?

Do you get blurred vision or itchy, burning eyes?

Results

The higher your score, the greater the potential toxic burden you may be carrying and the more you may benefit from a detoxification and cleansing program.

- *If you scored 20 or higher:* You will *significantly* benefit from detoxifying your body, which could lead to weight loss and improved health and vitality. It is strongly recommended that you look into different ways to detoxify the body.

- *If you scored between 5 and 19:* You will *likely* benefit from a detoxification program for improved health and vitality.

- *If you scored below 5:* You might actually be free of toxic overload in the body and living a very healthy, toxin-free life. Good for you!

Although our bodies have the ability to eliminate toxins, it's when the body gets overloaded with toxins that it stores them in fat cells. Fat cells don't get broken down very easily, so they literally weigh down the body and make it bigger. As toxins accumulate, we begin to experience health problems like allergies, migraines, major diseases, and fatigue/low energy.

The 10-Day Green Smoothie Cleanse is a truly health-transforming experience. Here is how you do it:

1. Each day you drink up to 60 ounces of green smoothies per day. Simply prepare your entire day's worth of green smoothies in the morning and pack it up to take with you. Keep it refrigerated as much as possible. Drink one-third every three to four hours throughout the day or sip on the smoothie as you get hungry.

2. You may snack on apples, celery, carrots, cucumbers, and other crunchy veggies throughout the day. Other high-protein snacks include unsweetened peanut butter, hard-boiled eggs, and raw or unsalted nuts and seeds (only a handful).

3. Drink at least eight glasses of water (64 ounces) per day as well as detox or herbal teas, as desired.

4. Perform one of the two methods for colon cleansing, as needed (see chapter 5).

5. DO NOT CONSUME refined sugar, meat, milk, cheese, liquor, beer, coffee, sodas/diet sodas, processed foods, fried foods, refined carbs (white bread, pastas, donuts, etc.)

Also, be sure to join our Facebook group to get support, encouragement, and tips from me and others at:

https://www.facebook.com/groups/Green.Smoothie.Cleanse/

So let's learn how to detox to jumpstart losing weight and getting healthy! Keep reading!

CHAPTER TWO

Why Green Smoothies?

*G*reen Smoothies are quickly taking the health world by storm! Green smoothies are surprisingly simple, consisting of raw organic fruit, raw organic leafy greens, and water. (The recommended fruit:greens ratio is 6:4.) Despite their simplicity, green smoothies provide a ton of nutritional benefits that lead to a healthier lifestyle. These benefits include weight loss, increased energy, reduction in food cravings, clearer skin, and much more.

Ten Great Reasons to Drink Green Smoothies

1. NUTRIENT-RICH: The ingredients in smoothies are all raw and thus more nutritious. The extremely high temperatures often used during cooking destroy many of the nutrients in our food. Green smoothies are loaded with beneficial vitamins, minerals, antioxidants, anti-inflammatory substances, phytonutrients, fiber, water, and more! They are also stuffed with chlorophyll, which is similar in structure to the hemoglobin in human blood. So drinking green smoothies is much like receiving a cleansing blood transfusion.

2. **WEIGHT LOSS.** If you are trying to lose weight, you will be pleasantly surprised to learn that green smoothies are an excellent way to do so. They have a high water content and are filled with green leafy veggies, which you can eat in abundance and still not gain weight. They also have a high fiber content that will help you stay full and reduce cravings.

3. **DETOXIFICATION.** Our body naturally tries to eliminate toxins, but overexposure to any of them will slow down the body's detoxification systems. The reality is that you can assist the body in detoxifying and eliminating toxins that cause weight gain and harm your health. You can and should detoxify and cleanse the body if you want to live better and live longer. After your body utilizes nutrients from the food you eat, it must dispose of the unused food particles and waste produced by the digestive process. Without proper and complete elimination, undigested food can back up and leave toxins and waste in your body. But thanks to green smoothies, you can get the fiber you need to cleanse your body, tone your digestive system, and eliminate toxins.

4. **VIBRANT, RADIANT HEALTH.** A healthy body is vibrant, full of energy and life! I believe that natural, healthy eating is the secret to inner and outer beauty. When you eat natural, raw foods, you simply look and feel better and younger. Once you eat in a manner that keeps your cells clean and healthy, you will begin to look radiant, despite your age. Human beings are designed to eat a diet primarily made up of fruits, vegetables, seeds, and nuts. With these types

of natural, healthy foods, our bodies flourish and receive all of the necessary nutrients to keep our bodies toxin-free and looking our most beautiful. When you start drinking green smoothies, one of the first places where you'll see changes is in the quality of your skin. Healthy eating and living will remove years from your face, eliminate wrinkles, fade age spots, and give you a "second youth." Your skin will become supple, and acne will clear up. Your eyes will become brighter and begin to sparkle. The dark circles and puffiness will diminish as will the yellowness in the whites of your eyes. On the inside of your body, your cells will become rejuvenated as well, causing your organs to function more efficiently.

5. **EASY TO DIGEST.** Green smoothies are much easier to digest and metabolize than solid food. Just because you "eat" the right amount of fruits and vegetables every day does not mean you are automatically getting all the nutrients necessary for your health and well-being. There are many people who cannot effectively digest solid whole food, so the nutrients from the food are not completely absorbed by the body. Green drinks, which are in a blended, liquid form, are far easier to metabolize. In fact, these delicious smoothies are so bio-available that their nutrients start to get absorbed by the body even while the smoothie is still in your mouth!

6. **IMPROVE DIGESTION.** Today's standard American diet (SAD) has created numerous digestive issues such as heartburn, acid reflux, colitis, Crohn's disease, and irritable bowel syndrome (IBS), just to

name a few. The root of most digestive issues is low production of hydrochloric acid in the stomach. If enough stomach acid isn't produced during digestion, much of the food we eat goes through the digestive tract largely undigested, creating gas, bloating, and other digestive disturbances. Once undigested food builds up as plaque on the intestinal lining, it sets the stage for disease. Processed foods, excessive gluten and proteins, fried foods, and other unhealthy fats are the main reasons behind these digestive issues. Since green smoothies are thoroughly blended, the majority of the work your digestive system would normally need to do is already done. Your body can then more easily extract the nutrients needed for optimum health.

7. HYDRATION: Staying hydrated gives you energy and helps ensure that your brain, muscles, digestive system, and immune system all work properly. Being dehydrated can be very dangerous. Drinking soda or coffee, eating processed foods, and smoking cigarettes all dehydrate the body. The best way to tell whether you are sufficiently hydrated is to check the color of your urine. If it is very pale, yellow, or clear, then you are properly hydrated. You do not want it to be a strong yellow color. It's easy to forget to drink water throughout the day because of our busy, hectic lives. Many don't like the taste of water, but it is essential to a healthy, functioning body. To improve the taste of water, just add in fresh-squeezed lemon juice. Green smoothies allow you to rehydrate your body thanks to their high water content.

8. **SIMPLY DELICIOUS.** The sweet taste of the fruit in the smoothie offsets the taste of the greens, making for a tasty and filling meal or snack. Many people who turn their noses up at green smoothies when they first see them become hooked after they taste them! Even children love the taste.

9. **EASY TO MAKE.** Preparation time is five minutes or less, and cleanup is quick and easy, too. If you place all of your ingredients in a plastic bag in the evening, all you'll need to do in the morning is toss them in the blender the next morning. After you finish blending, you simply rinse the blender and it's ready for the dishwasher. The storage, blending, and cleanup really take only five minutes a day.

10. **UNLIMITED NUMBER OF RECIPES.** There are over a hundred green smoothie recipes in this book and many more online with which you can experiment. That means your taste buds never have to get bored. There are so many possible fruit, greens, and liquid combinations that you can literally have a different recipe for each day of the year. I keep my favorite recipes on index cards so I can use them over and over again.

I could go on and on about the numerous health benefits of green smoothies, but you'll learn more of them as we go through this book. When you try them, you'll soon discover the wonderful health benefits yourself.

WHICH GREENS AND WHY?

Here's a list of the most popular greens to use in green smoothies. Keep in mind that they are in alphabetical order, not necessarily in order of the most nutritious.

- **Arugula:** Arugula is a great source of folic acid as well as vitamins A, C, and K, and provides a boost for bone and brain health. It has a zippy, peppery flavor.

- **Beet Greens:** Beet greens are the leafy tops to the beet vegetable. They are rich in vitamin K. They are known to help improve vision, help prevent Alzheimer's, and boost the immune system.

- **Bok Choy:** Bok choy is a Chinese cabbage that is mild tasting and crunchy. It is full of vitamins A, C, and calcium, as well as antioxidants.

- **Chard (aka Swiss Chard):** Chard is a green leafy vegetable that displays red stalks, leaf veins, and stems. It has a beet-like taste and a mild texture. It is known to help prevent cancers and is good for cleansing the digestive system.

- **Collard Greens:** Collards are green leafy vegetables that are nutritionally similar to kale but chewier and with a much stronger taste. They are a superior agent for binding to bile acids throughout the digestive tract, which makes them very good at lowering cholesterol.

- **Dandelion Greens:** Dandelion greens look like weeds in your lawn, but they are yet another great source of vitamins A and K. They help the digestion process and can help constipation issues because they are a natural laxative.

- **Kale:** Kale is lightweight with ruffled leaf edges. It is loaded with vitamins A, C, K, and more. It is known for lowering the risks associated with developing prostate, ovary, breast, colon, and bladder cancers.

- **Lettuce:** Lettuce has been a popular staple in salads since the time of the Ancient Egyptians. It contains essential amino acids and vitamins. Be sure to eat lettuces with dark green leaves to get the highest nutritional value. Romaine lettuce, in particular, has high levels of vitamin C, K, and A and is a good source of folic acid.

- **Mustard Greens:** Spicy mustard greens are effective in lowering cholesterol and provide a healthy dose of riboflavin, niacin, magnesium, and iron. They are a storehouse of phytonutrients that have many disease-preventing properties.

- **Parsley:** Parsley is rich in antioxidants, minerals, vitamins, and fiber and is known to help reduce aging and regulate blood sugar levels.

- **Spinach:** Perhaps the most beloved green leafy vegetable of them all, spinach is mild tasting and not as bitter as other greens. Its dark green leaves really pack a punch with high levels of omega-3s, calcium, magnesium, and vitamins A, C, E, and K. When most people start drinking green smoothies, they start with spinach!

- **Turnip Greens:** Turnip greens, although slightly bitter, are very flavorful. Turnip greens are effective at providing many numerous health benefits, but they stand out amongst other green leafy veggies in their ability to fight the development of cancerous cells.

Milder-Tasting Greens:

- Baby beet greens
- Baby bok choy
- Butter lettuce
- Carrot top greens
- Kale
- Romaine lettuce
- Spinach
- Swiss chard

Stronger-Tasting Greens:

- Arugula
- Collard greens
- Dandelion greens
- Mustard greens
- Radish tops
- Sorrel
- Turnip greens
- Watercress

HOW IS BLENDING DIFFERENT FROM JUICING?

Juices and smoothies both have their health benefits, but I feel that in most cases, blending provides a wider range of benefits than juicing. Smoothies have more fiber, fill you up better, and are both less expensive and less time-consuming to make.

Smoothies contain whole foods with loads of fiber. In juicing, the pulp is discarded and you lose essential fiber. The main argument for those who prefer juicing is that the absence of fiber provides easy absorption of nutrients straight into the bloodstream with little digestion required, and this allows the digestive system and body to heal. But fiber is critical for slowing the passage of food through the stomach and it keeps sugars from getting into the bloodstream too quickly. This helps regulate blood sugar and aids in weight control. Consuming greens in your smoothies helps to balance blood sugar, and the high fiber content of greens helps slow carbohydrate digestion.

Smoothies are more filling than juices, leaving us full and satisfied and less likely to overeat throughout the day. This is excellent news for those who wish to lose weight. It is very easy to replace a meal with a smoothie, and many do this for breakfast every day.

Smoothies are less expensive because it takes less fruit and vegetables to make a smoothie than it does to make the same size glass of juice. When we drink green smoothies, we are filled up longer so this also prevents us from needing to buy a lot of other food throughout the day.

Blending is faster than juicing and easier to clean up afterwards. To make juice, all the fruit and vegetables must be cut up small enough to fit into the juicer and then processed one piece at a time. To make a smoothie, the fruits and veggies can go into the blender all at once. Additionally, a juicer must be taken apart to be cleaned and then put back together, which requires a lot of time and cleanup. Blenders just require rinsing, with no parts to disassemble.

It's also easy to add superfoods, like maca or acai berries, to blenders as they will be blended through very evenly.

THE PROTEIN MYTH

Green smoothies that consist of 40 percent greens are a great source of protein. Greens provide protein in the form of amino acids, the building blocks of protein. These are easier for the body to utilize than complex proteins like those found in meats and other animal products. Greens supply ample amounts of amino acids, which provide us with all the protein we need.

When one eats foods that contain proteins, the digestive system has to break down the proteins into individual amino acids in order for the body to utilize them. The proteins found in animal products are extremely difficult to digest, and after being cooked, they're even harder for the body to break down and utilize. The body spends so much energy breaking down these proteins into amino acids that much of their nutritional value is rendered invaluable to the body.

If you feel you need additional protein because of a heavy workout, feel free to add protein powder in your blender to add to your green smoothie.

CHAPTER THREE

Getting Prepared

*A*re you ready for one of the biggest challenges of your life? The 10-Day Green Smoothie Cleanse will challenge you spiritually, mentally, and physically. It will transform your life in so many positive ways. You will learn so much about yourself and your eating habits. You will also learn to have a better relationship with food. The only way to attain a healthy relationship with food is to learn to love it and ensure that the food you put into your body loves you back: it fuels you, nourishes you, and supports your optimal health and vitality. During the 10-Day Green Smoothie Cleanse, you will give your body healthy, nutrient-rich foods that make you feel alive! Know that there will be times when you feel frustrated or feel like giving up, but if you stick with it, your body will reward you for your efforts. You will be truly amazed at the results!

The first four days will be the most challenging part of your experience. As your body adjusts from receiving its calories from whole foods, to the blended, nutrient-rich green smoothies, it will initially crave what you were used to eating. This is normal so allow your body to adjust during the first four days even though you may feel uncomfortable at times. After the first few days, your body will become satisfied with the green smoothies and the amazing nutrients in them. You will begin to feel energized and healthy, maybe for the first time in years.

Because you are eating only blended foods (green smoothies), raw fruits and vegetables, and raw unsalted nuts and seeds, you digestive system has to do less work. This gives your body a chance to cleanse, heal and do some much needed repair work.

What to Include in Your Green Smoothie

For the 10-Day Green Smoothie Cleanse, the only acceptable foods to add in your smoothies are green leafy vegetables, fruits and water. Please do not add any starchy vegetables such as sweet potatoes, beets, carrots or any other vegetables that are not leafy greens. Fruit is normally digested quickly, but when it's mixed with other starchy vegetables, the stomach will let the fruit sit while it digests the other foods that are in there. The fruit will begin to ferment which causes gas and bloating. To avoid this, only add green leafy veggies, fruits and water in the green smoothies during the 10-day cleanse.

Be sure to only use the darker varieties of green leafy vegetables as they provide chlorophyll and other important nutrients. Some examples of dark, leafy greens are kale, chard, spinach, baby salad greens, arugula, romaine lettuce, dandelion greens, beet greens, and collard greens. Organic produce is superior and important to use during the cleanse. If you can't find organic fruits and vegetables, wash off the pesticides and waxes as best you can. Waxes are pretty difficult to remove; in fact, they usually can't be removed by simply washing them. You need to purchase special cleansers from health food stores. Be sure to rinse the produce after you scrub off the wax. You can also reduce the toxic content of fruits and vegetables by soaking and scrubbing them in a tub of 10 percent white vinegar and then washing them off with water.

It is important to use spring or purified water in your green smoothies. Another option is alkaline water, which aids in detoxification and better hydration. Tap water is not recommended for use.

Preparing for Day 1

Before you begin, it is important to get mentally prepared for your new journey. Each day, remind yourself of the wonderful benefits of the 10-day cleanse. Tell yourself that you can do this and look forward to improving your energy and health in ways you never thought possible.

Begin each morning by drinking a few glasses of water to replenish what was lost overnight. Follow with a cup of detox tea which will provide cleansing support for your liver and kidneys. Feel free to add stevia, a natural sweetener, to your detox tea to enhance the taste. It is very important to drink a lot of water each day during the cleanse. Staying hydrated will help your body flush away the toxins that it releases during the cleansing process. Frequent urination and bowel movements should be expected during the first few days of the 10-day cleanse.

Take Your Measurements and Photos

Weigh yourself and take your measurements (bust, waist, and hips), and record these numbers along with the date. Some people will lose more weight while others will lose more inches, so you want to measure both! The majority of you (80%) will lose 10 to 15 pounds in 10 days on the full cleanse.

Next, take photos of your entire body and of your face close-up. This will enable you to see the physical changes that take place. Many times you will see a big difference in the whites of your eyes, along with less dark circles and puffiness. This way you can monitor your progress not just by the weight on the scale but how you look and feel overall.

This isn't just about weight loss... It's about getting healthy. So you want to monitor your energy, digestion, moods, mental clarity, and radiance of your skin! Get both the health and weight loss benefit! Don't let the scale become your enemy. Remember, weight loss can be up and down during a detox. But in the end, you'll still lose.

The Shopping List

I recommend buying fruits and veggies for five days at a time, so expect to shop twice during the ten-day cleanse. Here you'll see two lists—one for the first five days and the other for the final five days of the cleanse.

These lists assume you will follow the ten official Green Smoothie Cleanse recipes found in chapter 4.

Food for the First Five Days

- ☐ 6 apples
- ☐ 1 bunch grapes
- ☐ 20 ounces frozen peaches

- 20 ounces frozen blueberries
- 15 ounces frozen strawberries
- 10 ounces frozen mixed berries
- 6 ounces of mango chunks
- 3 bananas
- 1 bunch kale
- 20 ounces spinach
- 20 ounces spring mix greens
- Stevia sweetener (packets)
- Bag of ground flaxseeds (often in vitamin section)
- Fruit and veggies of your choice to munch on (such as apples, carrots, celery, etc.)
- Raw or unsalted nuts and seeds to snack on
- Detox tea (by Triple Leaf or Yogi brands)
- Sea salt (or any uniodized sea salt)
- OPTIONAL: Non-dairy/plant-based protein powder, such as RAW Protein by Garden of Life or SunWarrior protein

Food for the Last Five Days

- 20 ounces frozen mango chunks
- 20 ounces frozen peaches
- 20 ounces frozen pineapple chunks
- 10 ounces frozen mixed berries
- 6 ounces frozen blueberries
- 6 ounces frozen strawberries
- 2 apples

- [ ] 5 bananas
- [ ] 1 bunch kale
- [ ] 20 ounces spinach
- [ ] 20 ounces spring mix greens
- [ ] Fruit and veggies of your choice to munch on (such as apples, carrots, celery, etc.)
- [ ] Raw or unsalted nuts and seeds to snack on

CHAPTER FOUR

How to Do the 10-Day Green Smoothie Cleanse

The 10-Day Green Smoothie Cleanse is a truly health-transforming experience. You can choose to do a full cleanse or a modified cleanse.

The *full cleanse* consists of three smoothies, snacks, and water/tea for the entire ten days. This will provide the most health and weight-loss benefits, with an expected weight loss between ten and fifteen pounds.

The *modified cleanse* consists of two green smoothies (one for breakfast and one for lunch), with one healthy meal for dinner, snacks, and water/tea. The one healthy meal a day may consist of a salad, sautéed veggies, fish or chicken (grilled or baked).

The modified cleanse is a good plan with tremendous health benefits from the nutrient-rich smoothies. Weight loss may not be as dramatic, but you can expect to still lose between five and ten pounds in the ten days. The modified cleanse was designed for those unwilling or unable to stick with the full cleanse for ten days. It is also great for those who are not looking to lose a lot of weight but simply detox. If you're new to detoxing and want to gradually ease into the cleanse, this is a great option.

For either cleanse, you will avoid white sugar, meat, milk, cheese, liquor, beer, coffee, sodas/diet sodas, processed foods, fried foods and refined carbs (white bread, pastas, donuts, etc.) during the entire ten days.

FULL CLEANSE SUMMARY

1. **DRINK SMOOTHIES:** Each day, drink three green smoothies; one for breakfast, lunch and dinner. You can also sip on the smoothie throughout the day as you get hungry. It is important to drink a smoothie or eat a snack every three to four hours to keep your metabolism revved up. Each smoothie should contain about 12 to 16 ounces of liquid. Simply prepare your entire day's worth of green smoothies in the morning and pack it up to take with you. Keep it refrigerated as much as possible.

2. **EAT SNACKS:** You may snack on apples, celery, carrots, cucumbers, and other crunchy veggies that are appealing to you throughout the day. Other high-protein snacks include unsweetened peanut butter, hard-boiled eggs, and raw or unsalted nuts and seeds (only a handful).

3. **DRINK WATER AND DETOX TEA:** Drink at least eight glasses of water (64 ounces) per day, and drink detox or herbal teas as desired. Drink the detox tea first thing every morning as it aids the detox process by cleansing the detox organs—kidneys, liver, skin, etc.

4. **KEEP BOWELS MOVING:** Perform one of the two

methods for colon cleansing to ensure you have one to three bowel movements per day while detoxing. (See chapter 5.)

5. **DO NOT EAT** refined sugar, meat, milk, cheese, liquor, beer, coffee, sodas/diet sodas, processed foods, fried foods, refined carbs (white bread, pastas, donuts, etc.)

MODIFIED CLEANSE SUMMARY

1. **DRINK SMOOTHIES AND EAT ONE HEALTHY MEAL:** Each day, drink two green smoothies for breakfast and lunch, and eat one healthy meal for dinner. The one healthy meal may consist of a salad, sautéed veggies, and fish or chicken (grilled or baked). Any two meals can be used for the green smoothies, as long as you only have one healthy meal per day. Each smoothie should contain about 12 to 16 ounces of liquid. Simply prepare your entire day's worth of green smoothies in the morning and pack it up to take with you. Keep it refrigerated as much as possible.

2. **EAT SNACKS:** You may snack on apples, celery, carrots, cucumbers, and other crunchy veggies that are appealing to you throughout the day. Other high-protein snacks include unsweetened peanut butter, hard-boiled eggs, and raw or unsalted nuts and seeds (only a handful).

3. **DRINK WATER AND DETOX TEA:** Drink at least eight glasses of water (64 ounces) per day, and drink detox or herbal teas as desired. Drink the detox tea first thing every morning as it aids the

detox process by cleansing the detox organs—kidneys, liver, skin, etc.

4. **KEEP BOWELS MOVING:** Perform one of the two methods for colon cleansing to ensure you have one to three bowel movements per day while detoxing. (See chapter 5.)

5. **DO NOT EAT** refined sugar, red meat, milk, cheese, liquor, beer, coffee, sodas/diet sodas, processed foods, fried foods, refined carbs (white bread, pastas, donuts, etc.)

THE 10 DAYS OF RECIPES FOR THE 10-DAY GREEN SMOOTHIE CLEANSE

Here are the recipes for the ten days of the Green Smoothie Cleanse. You will have all of the ingredients on hand if you made use of the grocery-shopping list in chapter 3.

Use one recipe per day, as it will make enough for a full day's worth of smoothies. Be careful deviating from the recipes too much until after the detox/cleanse. These recipes were designed for detox, weight loss, better energy, and mental clarity. Try to stick to them as much as you can during the detox! You'll get better results. After the detox, get creative, add variety, and keep losing weight and getting healthy!

The unblended ingredients are about 72 ounces. Once blended, they will blend down to about 36 to 48 ounces, depending upon blender size and amount of water. Divide the total amount into thirds and drink each serving three to four hours apart or sip on the smoothie throughout the day whenever you feel hungry.

If you don't feel like drinking the entire day's worth of smoothie, then drink at least two of them to ensure your body gets the proper nutrition. It's important to drink a green smoothie or snack every three to four hours to keep your metabolism revved up. You will desire less food, but you still need to give your body fuel (smoothie or snack) every three to four hours.

IMPORTANT NOTE: If you have a full-size blender, like a Vitamix or Blendtec or something similar, the entire recipe can go into the blender at one time, as it easily holds 72 ounces of ingredients. However, if you have a smaller blender, like a Nutribullet or something similar, they hold only about 32 ounces, so you may need to divide the recipe in half and blend twice to avoid spillovers.

Day 1: Berry Green

3 handfuls spinach

2 cups water

1 apple, cored, quartered

1 cup frozen mangos

1 cup frozen strawberries

1 handful frozen or fresh seedless grapes

1 stevia packet (add more to sweeten, if necessary)

2 tablespoons ground flaxseeds

OPTIONAL: 1 scoop of protein powder

> Place leafy greens and water into blender and blend until mixture is a green juice-like consistency. Stop blender and add remaining ingredients. Blend until creamy.

Day 2: Apple Strawberry

3 handfuls spring mix greens

2 cups water

1 banana, peeled

2 apples, cored, quartered

1½ cups frozen strawberries

2 stevia packets (add more to sweeten, if necessary)

2 tablespoons ground flaxseeds

OPTIONAL: 1 scoop of protein powder

Place leafy greens and water into blender and blend until mixture is a green juice-like consistency. Stop blender and add remaining ingredients. Blend until creamy.

Day 3: Apple Berry

1 handful spring mix greens

2 handfuls spinach

2 cups water

1½ cups frozen blueberries

1 banana, peeled

1 apple, cored and quartered

1 packet stevia

2 tablespoons ground flaxseeds

OPTIONAL: 1 scoop of protein powder

Place leafy greens and water into blender and blend until mixture is a green juice-like consistency. Stop blender and add remaining ingredients. Blend until creamy.

Day 4: Berry Peachy

2 handfuls kale

1 handful spinach

2 cups water

2 apples, cored, quartered

1½ cups frozen peaches

1½ cups frozen mixed berries

2 packets stevia

2 tablespoons ground flaxseeds

OPTIONAL: 1 scoop of protein powder

> Place leafy greens and water into blender and blend until mixture is a green juice-like consistency. Stop blender and add remaining ingredients. Blend until creamy.

Day 5: Peach Berry Spinach

3 handfuls spinach

2 cups water

1 cup frozen peaches

1 handful fresh or frozen seedless grapes

1½ cups blueberries

3 packets stevia to sweeten

2 tablespoons ground flaxseeds

OPTIONAL: 1 scoop of protein powder

Place spinach and water into blender and blend until mixture is a green juice-like consistency. Stop blender and add remaining ingredients. Blend until creamy.

Day 6: Pineapple Spinach

2 cups fresh spinach, packed

1 cup pineapple chunks

2 cups frozen peaches

2 bananas, peeled

1½ packets stevia

2 cups water

2 tablespoons ground flaxseeds

OPTIONAL: 1 scoop of protein powder

Place spinach and water into blender and blend until mixture is a green juice-like consistency. Stop blender and add remaining ingredients. Blend until creamy.

Day 7: Pineapple Berry

2 handfuls spring mix greens

2 handfuls spinach

1 banana, peeled

1½ cups pineapple chunks

1½ cups frozen mango chunks

1 cup frozen mixed berries

3 packets stevia

2 cups water

2 tablespoons ground flaxseeds

OPTIONAL: 1 scoop of protein powder

> Place leafy greens and water into blender and blend until mixture is a green juice-like consistency. Stop blender and add remaining ingredients. Blend until creamy.

Day 8: Spinach Kale Berry

2 handfuls kale

2 handfuls spinach

2 cups water

1 apple, cored, quartered

1 banana, peeled

1½ cups frozen blueberries

2 packets stevia

2 tablespoons ground flaxseeds

OPTIONAL: 1 scoop of protein powder

Place leafy greens and water into blender and blend until mixture is a green juice-like consistency. Stop blender and add remaining ingredients. Blend until creamy.

Day 9: Apple Mango

3 handfuls spinach

2 cups water

1 apple, cored, quartered

1½ cups mangoes

2 cups frozen strawberries

1 packet stevia

2 tablespoons ground flaxseeds

OPTIONAL: 1 scoop of protein powder

Place spinach and water into blender and blend until mixture is a green juice-like consistency. Stop blender and add remaining ingredients to blender. Blend until creamy.

Day 10: Pineapple Kale

2 handfuls kale

1 handful spring mix greens

2 cups water

1½ cups frozen peaches

2 handfuls pineapple chunks

2 packets stevia

2 tablespoons ground flaxseeds

OPTIONAL: 1 scoop of protein powder

Place leafy greens and water into blender and blend until mixture is a green juice-like consistency. Stop blender and add remaining ingredients. Blend until creamy.

CHAPTER FIVE

JJ's Personal Tips for Success

Here are a few tips that will help you be successful!

Join our Facebook group. Get support, encouragement, and tips from me and others at:

https://www.facebook.com/groups/Green.Smoothie.Cleanse/

Blender size will make a difference. Use a high-speed blender (around 1000 watts), such as Vitamix, Blendtec, or Nutribullet. With a high-speed blender, you should only have to blend for 30 seconds to one minute until your smoothie is creamy and smooth. However, if you have a regular blender, then plan on doubling the blending time to one to two minutes.

Add protein to your shake. Extra protein is not mandatory for this cleanse, which is why you will see it listed as optional. However, as a nutritionist, I recommend adding one scoop of protein per day because it will help keep you feeling full longer and your metabolism revved up. The protein can make the smoothie taste slightly pasty, so try the smoothie first without it and then add the protein to see if it is palatable to you. Since you will be avoiding dairy (cow's milk) during the cleanse, be sure you use a non-dairy, plant-based protein powder, such as rice, soy, or hemp protein, and not whey protein powder, which is made from cow's milk. My favorite brands are RAW Protein by Garden of Life, Sunwarrior's Protein Blend, or Rainbow Light's Acai Berry Blast Protein Energizer. However, there are other quality options also. Other great sources of protein include hard-boiled eggs, raw or unsalted nuts and seeds, especially chia seeds or flaxseeds, and unsweetened peanut butter.

Chew your smoothies. Try to go through the chewing motion as much as possible, as the saliva in your mouth starts the digestive process. So, in as much as you can remember, try "chewing" your smoothie. This will also help minimize gas and bloating.

Expect your weight to fluctuate. While detoxing, you may gain on some days, while other days you may lose weight. This is perfectly normal. Weight fluctuates due to three things in the body: muscle, fat, and water. Muscle weighs the most—that's why you can work out and build muscle and thereby gain weight. But you're actually making progress by building muscle because it will help you burn fat all day long. For women, water is the biggest culprit, due to our hormones.

Many of us gain five to ten pounds of water weight during our cycle. For some, excess salt/sodium causes water to be trapped under the tissues in the body, making us weigh more and look bloated and puffy! So don't sweat it if your weight loss is a little up and down. When it's up every week, week after week, then you know you have a problem! Also, look into getting a Tanita scale—it will tell you your weight and percentage of muscle, fat, and water in the body. This is helpful for people who work out!

Remove the stems from your greens. Many greens such as kale, collards, etc., come packaged without the stems, but if not, be sure to destem the stalks from all green veggies, as they alter the taste quite a bit. I like to buy my greens already destemmed.

Rotate your greens. All greens have certain types of alkaloids in them. Now, these alkaloids are in very small, unharmful amounts, but if you continually take in the same type of greens week after week, you can get a buildup of that type of alkaloid and suffer serious health issues. The easiest way to avoid this is to rotate your greens. One week, buy spinach, the next week, kale, the next week, romaine lettuce. Or you can buy two greens for one week and then two different greens the following week. The goal is to rotate different greens into your smoothies each week. There are plenty of green leafy veggies to choose from.

Use ripe fruit. Ripe fruit is more digestible because of the live enzymes in it. If you buy it less than ripe, allow it to get ripe before you use it in the blender.

Use frozen fruit. Feel free to use frozen fruit instead of fresh fruit. Frozen fruit is cheaper and has just as much, if not more, of the nutritional value of fresh fruit. Also, fresh fruit can go bad within a few days, but you won't have this problem with frozen fruit.

Add ice. If all your fruit is fresh, use ice in place of the water to ensure the smoothie is cold.

Make it taste good. The recipes can be slightly altered to taste. So feel free to add more ice or water if your smoothie is too thick for your taste. Also, feel free to add more stevia to sweeten, if necessary. Stevia is a natural herbal sweetener that won't cause blood sugar spikes. You can add more fruit to sweeten as well. It's important that the smoothie taste good to you so you will continue with the cleanse.

Drink plenty of water. Ideally, drink 64 ounces per day, as it helps to flush out toxins. If you're drinking enough water, you will urinate frequently when you begin this detox, which is normal and a good thing!

Drink herbal and detox teas. Herbal teas are an important addition to your cleanse. Not only will herbal teas help you feel less hungry, they can also aid in the detoxification process. Good herbal teas to include are chamomile, peppermint, green tea, dandelion root, ginger, milk thistle, sarsaparilla, and ginseng. However, my favorite brand designed specifically for cleansing is a Detox Tea by Triple Leaf and Yogi brands. Be sure to add stevia to taste.

Diabetics, use low-sugar fruit! People with diabetes have to closely monitor their sugar intake with each meal. The biggest concern for diabetics is the natural sugar content in green smoothies. It is recommended that diabetics or those who suffer with candida use only low-sugar fruits such as apples, grapefruits, lemons, limes, cherries, strawberries, cranberries, raspberries, goji berries, and blueberries. Moderate-sugar fruits include peaches, oranges, pears, apples, pomegranates, and plums. The high-sugar fruits are apricots, melons, kiwis, mangos, papayas, pineapples, bananas, dates, figs, raisins, and grapes. Be sure to monitor your blood sugar throughout the day to see that the numbers are stable! And, of course, get your doctor's permission before you proceed with the cleanse.

Keep your bowels moving. Your bowels should move one to three times per day, optimally, and never less than once a day. It is absolutely imperative that your bowels move toxins out of your system while cleansing. If you haven't had a bowel movement in over 24 hours, there are two methods to get your bowels moving. Method 1: Use the saltwater flush (SWF), which involves drinking uniodized sea salt with water. To tolerate the taste, you can drink two teaspoons of sea salt in eight ounces of water to make it go down and then follow immediately with three more 8-ounce glasses of water. Do this first thing in the morning while you have an empty stomach, and you will have several bowel movements within thirty minutes to an hour. Method 2: One product that really works wonders at getting at the old fecal matter in your colon is Mag07, which I highly recommend. Take three to four pills at bedtime and you can look forward to a heavy bowel movement in the morning. Many of my clients use Mag07 for regular colon cleansing.

Don't starve yourself. Be sure to snack between smoothies. This is not a starvation diet. Great snacks are high-protein ones, such as unsweetened peanut butter or hard-boiled eggs. You can also snack on uncooked veggies, fruits, and unsalted or raw nuts and seeds (just a handful).

Go easy on the fruit. Yes, they hide the greens, but too much fruit will spike your blood sugar, cause headaches, and give you an uncomfortable feeling under your skin. Pick a new fruit each day, or if you must, add several different fruits in very small doses. Although it's natural sugar, your body doesn't know the different between nature's sugar and high fructose, other than its addictive properties! So don't overdo it on the fruit!

Detox family and friends. Sometimes you need to detox your emotions as well as your body by withdrawing from family and friends who discourage you, tell you "you can't do it" or "you're not ready to do it," blah blah blah! If there is negative talk coming from some people in your life, I would encourage you to limit the amount of time you spend with them. We all have enough negative thoughts on our own without people adding to them! Don't gravitate to people who tell you you can't do something. Know that when you start this cleanse, you will want to give up. It's normal. But I know that sometimes the only way to grow in life is to be uncomfortable. How else do you grow mentally, spiritually, and physically? When you cheat or mess up, it's no big deal. I guarantee you that if you cheat a little bit one day on the cleanse, you are still eating better than you've been eating most days prior to the cleanse. We call that progress! You are right where you're supposed to be on this journey! Uncomfortable, irritable, doubtful, cranky. And then one day, the joy, the energy, and the feeling of accomplishment settles in. Don't you want that feeling?

Prepare to be uncomfortable. For the first few days, you will feel hungry and irritable. Snack until your body adjusts to less food. You can snack to get rid of the hunger. However, if you snack all day, you will not lose as much weight. But don't worry about that. You have to focus on getting your body through this process if you stand any chance of breaking unhealthy eating habits. The body has the natural ability to maintain your ideal weight if you focus on getting healthy. As the days go on, you will want less food and will learn to eat in moderation. You are training your body to have better eating habits. So go through the process, be uncomfortable from time to time, and let your body reward you for it in the end. Many of us eat out of habit and boredom—that's called emotional hunger, not physical hunger. This is a perfect time to learn the difference between the two.

Follow the ten recipes provided for the cleanse. I encourage you to follow the ten specific recipes as they are listed in this book. The ten days of recipes are designed for detox and weight loss. The ten recipes are nutritionally balanced with proteins, carbs and healthy fats. Don't substitute the water with other liquids. As an example, coconut water may make a smoothie taste better, but it is also high in natural sugar. This means that if you're trying to break a sugar addiction, coconut water will slow the process of breaking that addiction. After the ten days, as you continue on your green-smoothie journey, feel free to add other fruits, oils, veggies, and some of the superfoods listed in this book. You have a whole lifetime to get creative with green smoothie recipes.

Build a green-smoothie recipe box. Every time you drink a smoothie, write the recipe down on an index card and give it a score on a scale of 1 to 10. That way you'll build up a store of recipes that you love. In the Appendix and FAQs section, there is a list of websites with tons of great recipes you'll want to try after the ten-day cleanse.

Focus on getting healthy, and the weight loss will follow. If you're doing the cleanse for fast weight loss, you're totally missing the point! Getting on the scale every day is a waste of time. You will not lose pounds every day, and guess what, some days you may actually gain weight because your body is adjusting during the cleansing process. So prepare yourself for the journey! Don't waste time being discouraged by the scales. Don't let the scales become your enemy! Most folks lose between 10 and 15 pounds on the full cleanse. Sure, a few have lost less than nine, but some have lost as much as 20! However, the focus is on healthy eating and healthy living. Look at your energy level, skin, sleep, and digestion. If you focus on fast weight loss, you'll be on a diet for life. I'm done with dieting! Ninety-five percent of people who lose weight on a fad diet gain it back in three to five years. You need to change your eating habits for life. You will re-train your taste buds to desire healthier foods. Embrace a lifestyle change where you desire and crave healthy foods, where you never have to count calories and serving sizes, and you truly won't have to diet again! Focus on getting healthy, and the weight loss will follow.

Expect detox symptoms. This is important to understand, and I explain in detail what you can expect in the next section. Please read on.

Expect and Welcome Detox Symptoms

You may experience detoxification symptoms, and their severity will depend on how toxic you were to begin with. You should expect and welcome detox symptoms because, although they can be unpleasant, they are signs of progress.

Typical detox symptoms include the following:

- *Headaches, pains, nausea.* If you drink a lot of coffee, expect headaches during the first few days. You may also experience physical aches and joint pains or even nausea. If headaches get really bad, take a painkiller, as long as you have no health issues with these products.

- *Cravings.* As your body detoxifies, it craves foods it was used to eating, such as meat, dairy, sugar, and caffeine. Cravings may last for several hours or several days, but they will begin to decrease as your body gets rid of its toxic overload.

- *Fatigue.* Allow time to rest during this detoxification phase, as eliminating toxins will drain you and make you feel exhausted. Just take it easy and rest.

- *Muscle aches.* You may feel achy, as if you're catching a cold or flu. You may get a release of some mucus, so expect a runny nose.

- *Skin rashes.* Skin rashes, or even acne, are signs that your body is excreting toxins through your skin, which is the body's largest organ of elimination. By doing colonics, the saltwater flush, or taking the colon-cleansing herbs (like Mag07), you can minimize the rashes and breakouts.

- *Irritability.* Not eating some of your favorite foods will make you feel irritable and bored, so expect to be a little cranky. This is a good time to avoid social events as well.

If the detox symptoms are too strong, simply follow these guidelines:

1. ***Change the ratio of fruit to vegetables.*** Start with 30% greens to 70% fruit and work your way up to more greens and less fruit over time.

2. ***Hydrate.*** Drink lots of water to help with the cleansing process.

3. ***Ease gradually into the full cleanse.*** On your first day, have a green smoothie for breakfast and eat light, healthy meals for lunch and dinner (big salads). Remember to still avoid sugar, meats, dairy, etc. On your second day, have green smoothies for breakfast and lunch but a light healthy meal, such as a salad, for dinner. By the third day, you should be ready to resume with green smoothies all day. If not, just switch to the modified cleanse for the remainder of the cleanse period.

CHAPTER SIX

How to Continue Losing Weight After the 10-Day Cleanse

Congratulations on taking control of your health by caring for your body and feeding it what it needs to be slim, healthy, and vibrant! You will reap the rewards now and continue to enjoy a lifestyle of optimal health and happiness. Be sure to always make time to nourish your inner spirit and soul by giving your body the rest and relaxation it needs to stay strong and healthy. You have given yourself a wonderful gift of optimal health and wellness.

Breaking the Cleanse

Do not go right back into eating whole foods right after the cleanse!

Now that you have not been eating your normal diet for a time and your body has been cleansing, it is of utmost importance that you slowly begin adding whole foods back into your diet. You may feel tempted to eat a lot, but this can be very damaging to your system. Take at least three days to reintroduce whole foods. Salads are a good way to start. Make delightful salad dressings to please your palate.

Continue drinking your smoothies and listen to your body to see what foods work well for you.

In the first two days after the cleanse, drink a green smoothie for breakfast and have a salad or sautéed veggies for lunch and dinner. The goal is to eat very light. Going back to eating whole foods too quickly can make you feel bloated and nauseous. Trust me! This happened to me—I was really bloated! Ugh!

The third day after the cleanse, you should be able to have one green smoothie for breakfast and light meals (salads and lean, healthy meats such as fish or chicken) for lunch and dinner. By the fourth day, you should be able to eat whole foods easily, but keep your meals light and healthy. You won't crave unhealthy foods at this point, so it should be fairly easy to do. It's a good habit to always start your day with a green smoothie for breakfast to maintain weight loss.

Even one green smoothie a day used as a replacement meal will put you on the road to permanent weight loss and better health. It will reawaken your metabolism and give you more energy.

You deserve to be happy, healthy, and fit! Whatever happened in the past, whatever bad eating choices you might have made, those need to remain in the past. Look to your future, keep moving forward, and make food choices that make you feel good inside.

Continuing to Lose Weight After the Cleanse

Normal weight loss of about one to two pounds per week is very healthy! This cleanse should give you a ten- to fifteen-pound jumpstart on your weight loss to get you motivated to continue!

To continue weight loss at about two pounds per week, drink two green smoothies a day and eat one clean, high-protein meal. To continue weight loss at about one pound per week, drink one green smoothie and have two clean, high-protein meals per day. See the appendix for a list of clean, high-protein recipes.

"Clean" foods are natural, whole, raw, or organic foods that the body can effectively digest and utilize for energy without leaving excess waste or toxins in the body. "Clean" foods include lean proteins, good carbs, and healthy fats.

Why have protein every time you eat? Protein counteracts the body's overreaction to carbohydrates, which causes insulin spikes and fat storage. Protein will help you feel full longer and thus help prevent overeating and food cravings. Protein will also help you build and maintain muscle mass, and we've learned that muscle naturally burns more calories than fat.

Following are ten examples of clean, high-protein meals:

1. Grilled salmon with a garden salad
2. Lean steak with sweet potatoes and veggies
3. Grilled salmon with quinoa and veggies
4. Tuna on a garden salad
5. Chicken or lean steak in a Caesar salad
6. Grilled halibut with stir-fried veggies
7. Baked chicken with baked sweet potato and sautéed veggies
8. Chicken stir-fry with brown rice
9. Lean sirloin steak with lima beans
10. Turkey chili

I don't recommend that anyone stay on the full cleanse for longer than two weeks straight. You should always give your body a break after a detox cleanse. This also keeps your metabolism revved up by mixing up the foods you eat each week. Although I don't recommend it, if you choose to do the full cleanse longer than two weeks, you have to deliberately add more protein to your diet and be sure to rotate or use different greens each week!

A diet of two smoothies plus a high-protein meal per day is very healthy and can be done every day for life. And don't be rigid about your smoothie ritual or you'll get bored. Some days you may feel like eating a hearty breakfast, so have your smoothies for lunch and dinner. Mix it up!

I would also encourage that you "get moving" even if you can't get to a gym. Examples would be to take the stairs instead of elevators, walk to get lunch, park as far as you can from the grocery store or mall and walk the remaining distance, etc. Exercise is great for overall health, and we should all do it! If you become more active, you will enhance both your weight-loss efforts and your overall health. And getting moving does not necessarily mean going to the gym.

If Weight Loss Stalls

If you begin to plateau and weight loss stalls (if two weeks have gone by and you've not lost any more weight), I know exactly what you have to do next: Check your hormones. If you have stubborn body fat that is not responding to healthy eating, then hormones are the likely culprit! In my bestseller *Lose Weight Without Dieting or Working Out*, I have two chapters titled "Correct Hormonal Imbalances" and "Stop Weight Gain During Perimenopause and Menopause" that explain the six hormones that cause weight gain by slowing your metabolism and preventing your body from losing weight.

It is essential to understand the role hormones play in how we gain and lose weight. Some hormones tell you you're hungry, some tell you you're full; some tell your body what to do with the food that is eaten, whether to use it as fuel for energy or store it as fat, which causes us to gain weight. Hormones are responsible for metabolizing fat. By controlling your hormones, you can control your weight.

Hormones affect how you feel, how you look, and, most important, how you maintain your weight and health. When your hormones are balanced properly, you will have great health, beauty, and vibrancy. When your hormones are imbalanced, you have mood swings, you crave unhealthy foods, and you feel sluggish and lethargic. Hormones are critical to weight loss, and balancing them will help you stay slim and healthy.

Weight Loss Tips: Weight Loss the Healthy, Natural Way

Eat a big salad daily. Include dark leafy greens and lots of colorful vegetables every single day.

Drink at least one green smoothie daily. This along with the salad will really add a lot of nutrition to your body and will stave off unhealthy cravings. You can add some protein, flaxseeds, spirulina, coconut oil, and bee pollen to it for an extra health boost.

Choose nutrient-rich foods, not empty calories. Eat foods high in vitamins, minerals, phytonutrients, fiber, and omega-3 fatty acids. Junk foods contain only nutritionally empty calories. You want your calories to provide you with nutritional benefits that will help you heal your body and maintain a permanently healthy weight.

Eat protein with every meal. Eat the protein before the carbohydrates or fats. You can also eat protein by itself. Protein-rich foods do not cause insulin spikes, and so are important clean and balanced foods. Whenever you eat a carbohydrate, eat some protein along with it. As a general guideline, the protein should be about half the amount of the carbohydrates. For example, if you have 30 grams of carbohydrates, then eat about 15 grams of protein along with it to prevent insulin spikes that cause excess fat to be stored in the body.

Avoid sugar, salt, and trans fat. These are the top three ingredients that cause weight gain. Try to avoid them at all costs. They have no nutritional value and are simply bad for your health. Salt causes bloating, swelling, and fluid retention. The good news on trans fat is that the FDA regulates it, and food manufacturers now have to list how much is in each serving when trans fat exceeds 0.5 grams per serving.

Limit red meat to two or three times per week. Red meat contains a lot of saturated fat, so try to limit your intake to two or three times a week. Instead, eat more protein from fish, poultry, and vegetables, such as brown rice, beans, and nuts, which contain good essential fats.

Eat at least 30 grams of fiber per day. Numerous studies have shown that high-fiber diets help you lose weight and protect against heart disease, stroke, and certain kinds of cancer.

Eat four to five times a day. You will lose weight more quickly if you eat four or five times a day as opposed to only three times. Try to eat every three to four hours and think in terms of three meals and two healthy snacks. Each time you eat, you stimulate your metabolism for a short period of time; thus, the more often you eat, the more you speed up your metabolism. Eating every two to three hours feeds your muscles and starves fat.

Buy organic as much as possible. Buy organic foods, which don't have chemical preservatives, food additives, hormones, pesticides, and antibiotics. Fresh organic foods are far less toxic than highly processed and packaged/frozen foods and leave less residue and waste in the body.

Drink more pure water. Water does an amazing job of detoxifying your body. The trick though is to not drink water with your meals. This will dilute your digestive juices and make digestion less efficient. Do not drink anything thirty minutes before you eat a meal, and then wait two hours after a meal to have a drink. It is amazing how much energy you will get from doing this. Also, sometimes thirst is disguised as hunger. So there is a good chance that when you drink water, that hungry feeling will go away.

Drink green tea. Try to make the switch from coffee to green tea, ideally a non-caffeinated brand if possible. Green tea is particularly helpful for reducing body fat and weight, stimulating digestion, and preventing high blood pressure. There are many wonderful benefits of drinking green tea, but as far as weight loss goes, it simply helps the body burn fat faster and more efficiently. Green tea is better than black tea or coffee because its caffeine works in a different way. Green tea makes the body's own energy use more efficient, thereby improving vitality and stamina without your having to experience the up-and-down effect typically experienced with caffeine. This is due to the large amount of tannins in green tea that ensure that the caffeine is taken to the brain in only small amounts, which harmonizes the energies in the body.

Don't give in to emotional hunger. You have to learn the difference between physical hunger and emotional hunger. If you feel the desire to eat, but you have just eaten within the last two hours, you may actually be looking for a way to change your mood. See if you can find something to occupy yourself for at least one hour. Set a timer and drink some water. Tell yourself that you will eat in one hour. This will set your mind at ease. Then find a way to stay occupied or a way to feel fulfilled for that hour.

Best and Worst Foods to Eat if You're Trying to Lose Weight

This chart will help you understand what foods to eat and which to avoid to help you reach your weight loss goals. If you want to accelerate your weight loss, focus on eating more foods on the left side of the chart.

TYPE	FOODS TO EAT (support weight loss)	FOODS TO AVOID (cause weight gain)
Meats	Bass, Calamari, Clams, Crabmeat, Catfish, Cod, Cornish hen, Flounder, Haddock, Halibut, Herring, Lobster, Oysters, Sardines, Scallops, Shrimp, Skinless Chicken, Turkey breast, Sole, Tilapia, Trout, Tuna, Turkey bacon, Wild Salmon	Bacon, Beef jerky, High fat meats like Prime rib, Porterhouse, Hot dogs, Pepperoni, Salami, Sausage
Veggies	All dark greens, Asparagus, Avocados, Broccoli, Brussels sprouts, Cabbage, Cauliflower, Carrots, Celery, Cucumbers, Collards, Garlic, Green Beans, Kale, Lettuce, Mushrooms, Olives, Onions, Parsley, Peas, Radishes, Red Peppers, Squashes, Sweet Potatoes, Spinach, Tomatoes, Yams, Zucchini	All vegetables are generally good for you; however if you're trying to lose weight, try to avoid eating white potatoes, red potatoes, corn, and plantains
Fruits	In general, all fruits are healthy for you. However, if you're trying to lose weight (or are diabetic), the best fruits to eat are low-sugar fruits, which include Blackberries, Blueberries, Cranberries, Grapefruits, Lemons, Limes, Passion Fruit, Raspberries, Strawberries	Canned fruits, dried fruits, and fruit snacks
Grains (breads, pasta, rice)	Barley, Brown rice, Bulgur, Buckwheat, Coconut Flour, Oats (steel-cut oats), Quinoa, Wild rice	Bagels, Donuts, White rice, White pasta, White bread, White flour

TYPE	FOODS TO EAT (support weight loss)	FOODS TO AVOID (cause weight gain)
Beans/ Legumes	Black-eye peas, Black beans, Butter beans, Fava beans, Garbanzo beans /Chickpeas, Green beans Kidney beans, Peas, Lentils, Lima beans, Navy beans/Pinto beans, White beans	Dried beans, Refried beans
Dairy	Egg whites, Eggs, Almond milk, Coconut milk, Goat's milk, Hemp milk, Oat Milk, Rice Milk, Non-dairy butter (vegan butter)	Regular (full-fat) Cow's milk, Cheese, Cottage Cheese, Cream Cheese, and Sour Cream; Condensed milk, Powdered milk, Powered eggs, Yogurt with fruit on the bottom
Nuts and Seeds	Raw and Unsalted Nuts and Seeds: Almonds, Brazil nuts, Cashews, Cedar nuts, Hazelnuts, Macadamia nuts, Peanuts, Pecans, Pistachios, Walnuts; Seeds: Chia seeds, Flaxseeds, Hemp seeds, Pumpkin seeds, Sesame seeds, Sunflower seeds. The next best are roasted and unsalted nuts and seeds.	Sugar-coated nuts and seeds
Oils	Avocado oil, Coconut oil, Extra-virgin Olive oil, Fish oil, Flaxseed oil, Sesame oil	Bacon fat, Chicken fat, Margarine, Hydrogenated oils (trans fats), Vegetable oils

TYPE	FOODS TO EAT (support weight loss)	FOODS TO AVOID (cause weight gain)
Sweeteners	Listed in order of the best sweetener if you want to lose weight: Stevia, Monk fruit, Xylitol, Agave nectar, Raw honey, Coconut palm sugar, Sugar alcohol	White sugar, High-fructose corn syrup, Brown rice syrup, Brown sugar, Dextrose, Fruit juice concentrate, Raw sugar
Spices & Seasonings	Apple cider vinegar, Black pepper, Cardamom, Cayenne pepper, Chili peppers, Cilantro, Cinnamon, Ginger, Parsley, Garlic, Nutmeg, Onion, Oregano, Rosemary, Sage, Saffron, Tamari, Thyme, Turmeric	Ketchup, Mayonnaise, MSG, Table salt, Worcestershire sauce
Snacks	Fresh Fruits & Veggies, Popcorn (lightly salted), Unsweetened peanut/cashew/almond butter, Organic unsweetened chocolate, Nuts and seeds, Hard-boiled eggs, Plain yogurt, Trail mix	Candy, Pies, Corn chips, Cookies, Donuts, Cakes, Ice cream, Pastries, Potato chips
Beverages	Distilled or Spring water, Alkaline water, Coconut water, Fresh-squeezed juices, Green tea, Black tea, Mint tea/Other Herbal teas	Sodas, Sports Drinks, Store-bought fruit juices, Mixed drinks, Beer
Cooking Methods	Baking, Broiling, Grilling, Poaching, Pressure cooking, Roasting, Sautéing, Steaming, Stir frying	Barbequing, Blackening, Burning or Charring, Deep frying, Pan frying

Superfood Additions for Smoothies

These are the nutritional powerhouses that can increase the amounts of fiber, vitamins, minerals, and other nutrients in your smoothies. You can add these after the 10-day cleanse, as you make green smoothies a part of your daily lifestyle.

— Acai berries: power-packed with antioxidants that slow the aging process

— Aloe vera: has anti-inflammatory, anti-bacterial, and antifungal properties

— Avocado: full of healthy fats

— Bee pollen: increases energy and stamina

— Brewer's (nutritional) yeast: great source of vitamin B-12

— Cayenne pepper: will improve circulation and opens up the arteries

— Chia seeds: make you feel full and helps with weight loss

— Raw chocolate: high in antioxidants to slow the aging process

— Coconut oil: fat-burning power food that is antiviral and antibacterial

— Flax oil: boosts immune system and has anti-inflammatory effects

— Ginger: powerful anti-inflammatory and digestive-function strengthening properties

— Gogi berries: high in antioxidants to slow the aging process

— Maca root: improves energy levels and endocrine health

— Pomegranate juice: lowers cholesterol and has other cardiovascular benefits

— Sprouts: provide lots of enzymes and they oxygenate the body

— Wheat germ (raw): helps with PMS/menopause symptoms and healthy skin and hair

— Wheatgrass juice (fresh or powdered): alkalizes cells and boosts energy levels

— Yogurt or kefir: helps with digestion and fights against bacterial infections

Remember: The 10-day cleanse is a detox/cleanse, *not* a diet! Be smart about weight loss. Be in it for the long haul, expect weight to fluctuate, and prepare for the journey. Normal weight loss of about one to two pounds per week is very healthy. If you have 30 pounds to lose, it will likely take you fifteen weeks to lose it, so focus and lock in for four months! You *will* achieve your goal! Focus on *getting healthy.* The weight loss will follow!

CHAPTER SEVEN

Five Detox Methods to Enhance Your Cleansing

Detoxifying the body and eliminating toxins can be accomplished through various detoxification methods. (I describe twelve ways to detox the body for weight loss and overall health in my book *Lose Weight Without Dieting or Working Out*.)

Everyone's toxic overload is different, and many factors come into play, such as your health status, weight, metabolism, age, and genetics. If you want to enhance your detoxification and cleansing, here are five methods to detox the body to support the cleansing process during or after the 10-Day Green Smoothie Cleanse.

1. Colonics
2. Liver cleansing
3. Saunas
4. Body brushing
5. Detox foot bath/foot pads

Colonics

Colonics, also known as colon hydrotherapy, is a method

used to remove waste and impacted fecal matter from the colon. The first modern colonic machine was invented about a hundred years ago. Today, colonics are performed by colonic hygienists or colon therapists.

Colonics work somewhat like an enema but involve much more water and none of the odors or discomfort. While you lie on a table, a machine or gravity-driven pump slowly flushes up to 20 gallons of water through a tube inserted into the rectum. The therapist may use a variety of water pressures and temperatures. While the water is in the colon, he or she may massage the abdomen. Then the therapist flushes out the fluids and waste through another tube. The therapist may repeat the process. A session may last up to an hour.

The average colon weighs about four pounds, but it is not unusual at all for colon cleansing to flush away as much as ten to twenty pounds of stagnant fecal matter. Your colon can hold a great deal of waste material that, when not eliminated, putrefies, adding to the toxic load of your body. Many people with "pot bellies" may actually have several pounds of old, hardened fecal matter lodged within their colons. The process may actually cause you to experience some immediate weight loss.

It is a common misconception that doing a colonic will rid your body of all the good and bad bacteria. If you decide to do a colonic, it will rinse out good bacteria in your colon—but just temporarily. After you flush out everything, the good bacteria with the bad, you want to replace the good bacteria, the probiotics. Your body will replenish the good bacteria within twenty-four hours, unless you are extremely unhealthy or weak. However, you should always take a probiotic supplement after a colonic to replenish the good bacteria right away. A good colon therapist will always provide you with probiotics (good bacteria) at the end of your colonics session.

If you choose to research colonics and decide to include them as part of your detoxification process, you probably want to go at least once a week for up to six weeks, particularly when you first begin aggressively detoxifying the body. That is because you are drawing out toxins in the body, and if they are not eliminated quickly, they can cause detox symptoms that become uncomfortable. One rule of thumb as to whether to do a colonic is determined by how frequent your bowel movements are. If your body is managing the toxins and waste well through normal daily bowel movements (one to two per day), then you probably don't need to have a colonic. If your bowel movements are less frequent than once a day, it may be a good idea to do a colonic to get your bowels moving more frequently.

There are no major drawbacks to a properly administered colonic by a trained colon hydrotherapist. You don't need to be concerned about the safety of colonics as long as they're done with a certified colon therapist on a good-quality machine.

Check Your Poop to Evaluate Your Health

Here is another simple way to evaluate your health. As an example, bowel movements (BMs) that are black or reddish indicate potential health problems. Thin BMs suggest that more fiber is needed in the diet or there is some type of imbalance in the digestive tract. If you have chronic constipation and your BMs are rock solid, this may be an indication that your liver is overworked. If you experience chronic constipation or difficult bowel movements for an extended period of time, you should seek medical advice.

Your bowel movements will help you understand what's going on with your body. Healthy bowel movements should:

- Occur two to three times a day and definitely no less than once per day.

- Should not have a strong, foul odor.

- Should be medium brown in color, shaped like a banana, about the width of a sausage.

- Should float, not sink right to the bottom of the toilet.

Liver Cleansing

The one secret to losing weight and keeping it off is to keep the liver healthy and operating at peak performance. The liver (also known as the fat-burning organ) is the number-one secret weapon to weight loss. The liver is responsible for breaking down, eliminating, and neutralizing toxins in the body and breaking down fats in the body. Therefore, it is essential that we cleanse the liver to improve the body's detoxification capabilities and to help the body metabolize and burn fats.

When your liver functions efficiently, it is much easier for you to lose weight. The liver has to perform well enough to eliminate the toxins that are causing fat cells in the body. If you have body fat accumulation, especially around the waist and midsection (i.e., belly fat), it suggests that your liver may not be functioning properly or as efficiently as it could. To lose this excess weight, you have to detoxify and cleanse the liver, which leads to not only a slimmer waistline but also a thinner body.

One easy way to cleanse the liver is to take herbs/supplements, such as milk thistle, dandelion root, and burdock. These herbs are all-natural and very effective at liver detoxification. You'll find that many products on the market combine these herbs into one supplement so that you can achieve the best results. As you look for products to help you cleanse your liver, be sure to only use those that are all-natural and gentle on the body. My favorite two liver-cleansing supplements are Liver Rescue by Healthforce and Livatone Plus by Dr. Sandra Cabot.

Additionally, an inexpensive liver-cleansing option is to drink one to two tablespoons of apple cider vinegar in eight ounces of water every morning and night. Do this for two to three weeks or continue until your sluggish liver symptoms have improved. My favorite brand is Bragg Apple Cider Vinegar.

Completing a liver cleanse can be a positive and rejuvenating experience that yields numerous health benefits. As you improve liver health, you increase your body's ability to detoxify itself, improve its fat-burning capabilities, and achieve optimum health.

Saunas

The skin is the largest organ of elimination for the body, and a sauna helps you sweat out toxins from the body. Why I love the sauna is that I'm all about things that have a health benefit while providing a beauty benefit. You can kill two birds with one stone. You release toxins, burn calories, and come out with glowing skin. I had a client that learned from my teleseminars about saunas and found that by sweating out her toxins in the sauna, her acne cleared up; this was due to her sweating out the toxins as opposed to them being released through the skin, causing acne and other rashes.

If you want to know how healthy someone is, sometimes you can just look at his or her skin and tell. If someone has clear, radiant skin, there's a good chance he or she is very healthy; breakouts, puffiness, or dry skin indicate that the body is having some health problems. Experts say that a sauna session can do more to clean, detoxify, and simply "freshen" your skin than anything else. I personally love getting in the sauna.

Benefits of the Sauna:

- **Weight loss.** In a sauna, you can burn 300 to 500 calories in fifteen to twenty minutes, almost equivalent to one to two hours of brisk walking or one hour of exercise. Saunas works positively on metabolism, increasing its speed and intensity, which in turn results in weight loss.

- **Elimination of toxins.** The steam in a steam sauna opens up the pores, allowing the skin to sweat out toxins that can cause illness. Perspiration is how the body purges itself of toxins and impurities.

- **Cure for illnesses.** The heat of the steam causes the body's temperature to rise, which can help kill any virus, bacteria, fungus, or parasite in the body.

- **Improved skin.** The steam hydrates and moisturizes

the skin, making steam saunas particularly beneficial to people with dry skin.

- *Strengthened immune system.* The high temperature of a steam sauna causes an artificial fever, which sends a "wake-up call" to the immune system and increases an individual's white blood cell count.
- *Relaxed muscles.* The heat from the steam warms and relaxes tense muscles. This relaxation helps to reduce stress levels, revive mental clarity, and improve overall physical and emotional health.

For a steam sauna, you sit in moist heat for fifteen to twenty minutes. Follow that with a quick shower to wash off all of the toxins that have been flushed from your skin to feel truly refreshed.

Another type of sauna is an infrared sauna, which produces what is known as radiant heat. The heat of an infrared sauna also penetrates more deeply without the discomfort and draining effect often experienced in a conventional steam sauna. An infrared sauna produces two to three times more sweat volume, and due to the lower temperatures used (110 to 130 degrees), it is considered a safer alternative for those at cardiovascular risk. It accelerates the removal of toxic wastes and chemicals that are stored and lodged in the fatty tissues of the body. The sweating caused by deep heat helps eliminate dead skin cells and improves skin tone and elasticity. The heat produced in infrared saunas is extremely helpful for various skin conditions, including acne, eczema, and cellulite. Another benefit of the sauna is that you burn calories. Studies have shown that you can burn 600 calories in thirty minutes in an infrared sauna. Whichever you prefer, steam or infrared sauna, both can be dehydrating, so it is important to hydrate properly before and after a sauna.

A few of my personal tips for using a sauna:

- It is important to try out different types of saunas (steam, infrared, and oxygen steam sauna). You can make appointments at spas to see which type of sauna you like the best.

- You might want to invest in a home steam sauna. I bought one through Amazon.com for about $200, which is a lot cheaper than going to the spa every week.

- Sitting in the sauna one to two times per week is ideal for getting the best results.

- You will need to drink water before *and* after you get into the sauna. I drink coconut water after my sauna because it is super hydrating.

- If you have heart issues, sensitive skin, or asthma, or if you are pregnant, you should not sit in a sauna until you have checked with your doctor.

Body Brushing

Body brushing (also known as dry brushing) is done with a natural boar-bristle brush, which can be found in health food stores, Whole Foods, or Trader Joe's. Dry brushing on a regular basis lightens the burden on the liver by helping to remove excess waste in the body. Dry brushing stimulates the lymphatic system, which is a secondary circulatory system underneath the skin that rids the body of toxic wastes, bacteria, and dead cells. By body brushing, you move the toxins along and out of the body for elimination. By brushing the body from head to toe with the dry brush, focusing on the lymphatic drainage regions, like behind the knee, you'll improve the efficiency of the whole lymphatic system.

Firm, gentle brush strokes across the skin will improve your blood circulation, clean out clogged pores, and enable your body to remove toxins faster. Body brushing removes dead skin layers and encourages cell renewal for smoother skin. If the liver is the fat-burning organ, then the lymph system can be called a fat-processing system. So cleansing the liver and lymphatic system are key to weight loss and diminishing cellulite.

To effectively use the body brush, remove your clothes and begin brushing the soles of the feet. Next, brush from the ankles to the calves, concentrating on the area behind the knees, using long upward, firm strokes toward the heart. Then brush from the knees to the groin, the thighs, and the buttocks. If you're a woman, make circular strokes around your thighs and buttocks to help mobilize fat stores, such as cellulite. (Dry brushing actually helps to diminish cellulite.) Then brush the torso, avoiding the breasts. Finally, make long strokes from the wrists to the shoulders and underarms. The entire process should take no more than three to five minutes and will leave your skin feeling totally invigorated. The best times to brush are in the morning before showering or at night before bed.

Detox Foot Pads/Detox Foot Bath

Detox foot pads are a quick and easy way to rid the body of toxins. You put the pads on the bottoms of your feet overnight as you sleep. The ingredients in the detox foot pads are said to pull impurities and toxins out of your system during the night while you sleep. In the morning, you remove the pads from your feet and discard them. They are helpful with aches, pains, sore muscles, joint pains, swelling, and bloating.

The detox foot bath (ionic foot bath) works by soaking your feet in a warm saltwater solution made up of many different toxin-drawing ingredients. The ionic activity in the water shoots through your body fat and is supposed to draw the toxins out through the hundreds of pores in your feet. Thirty minutes is the average time for a detox foot bath, which costs a little more than the foot pads ($15 vs. $60 for a detox foot bath). A detox foot bath is said to make joint movement easier in the knees and elbows. It's an alternative-medicine option for people who suffer headaches and chronic joint and bone pain. A detox foot bath is very simple and extremely relaxing! If you want to get a detox foot bath, it is typically offered as a spa service under the name of Aqua Chi Foot Bath. For detox foot pads, my favorite brand is BodyRelief Foot Pads, which really helps me with joint aches and pains.

CHAPTER EIGHT

Frequently Asked Questions (FAQs)

Here are some of the most frequently asked questions about the 10-Day Green Smoothie Cleanse.

What if I'm too challenged with making it the entire ten days?

If this seems too big of a challenge, no worries. You may customize your experience by doing a five- or seven-day cleanse. However, you should take one day at a time and see how you feel after five days, seven days, and ten days.

Should I take my medications during the cleanse?

I am not a medical doctor, so you should talk to your doctor prior to starting the cleanse. I would personally never stop taking any medications prescribed by a doctor. However, the choice is yours.

Are there any supplements that are important to take?

Whether or not you continue to take your current vitamin supplements during the cleanse is up to you. I prefer not to take vitamin supplements when I cleanse.

Why are the greens chunky and not blended well?

Place only the leafy greens and the water into the blender and blend until the mixture is a green juice-like consistency. Then stop the blender and add the remaining ingredients. Blend again until the whole smoothie is a creamy consistency.

Can I exercise while doing the cleanse?

Exercising while on the cleanse is beneficial. However, if you feel really fatigued, rest! Listen to your body, and if it wants to rest, please do so. The best types of exercises are brisk walking or yoga. Keep things simple during a detox.

If you do not currently exercise regularly (this would be me!), start small. Take a fifteen-minute walk today and gradually increase your time over the next ten days. It is always best not to just dive right in and make yourself take an hour walk when you are not accustomed to exercising.

How long will my smoothie keep?

It is always ideal to drink your smoothie the same day you blend it to ensure you get maximum nutrition from it. However, if you are busy or for some other reason can't make them fresh, then they can keep extremely well for up to two days in the refrigerator. A glass jar with a lid is ideal to safely store your smoothies. Covering your green smoothies with a tight lid minimizes oxidation and absorption of other smells from the refrigerator. Additionally, making the smoothies the night before is okay if it helps you stay on track.

How many snacks can I have per day and in what serving sizes?

Don't think *diet*, think *detox cleanse*, so calories and serving sizes are not the focus. There are no hard and fast rules. But you should snack in moderation when you're hungry. Trying to eat by counting calories and serving sizes won't create a lifestyle change. You'll just be on a diet for life. I don't know about you, but I'm done with dieting! Ninety-five percent of people who lose weight on a fad diet gain it back in three to five years. So, you're changing your eating habits for life, retraining your taste buds to desire and crave healthier foods! Having said all that, the one caution I would give is on nuts and seeds. They are healthy fats but fats nonetheless. They can work against you if you eat too many. For a snack of nuts and seeds, think a handful!

How any ounces of the smoothie should I drink per day?

The unblended ingredients are about 72 ounces. Once blended, they will blend down to about 36 to 48 ounces depending upon blender size and amount of water used. You can drink three servings of 12 to 16 ounces each or feel free to sip on the smoothie throughout the day whenever you feel hungry.

What if I don't feel hungry or like drinking all three of the green smoothies for the day?

If you don't feel like drinking the entire day's worth of smoothies, then drink at least two of them to ensure your body gets the proper nutrition. It's important to drink a green smoothie or snack every three to four hours to keep your metabolism revved up. You will desire less food but must still give your body fuel.

How long can you stay on the full green smoothie cleanse?

I don't recommend the full cleanse be longer than two weeks straight. However, two green smoothies plus a high-protein meal per day is very healthy and can be done for life. If you choose to redo the full cleanse or do it for longer than two weeks, you have to deliberately add more protein into your diet and be sure to rotate or use different greens each week!

What if I feel like eating?

If you come to a point where you feel you would like to stop the cleanse, there are a few things to try. First, know this feeling will pass. Try making yourself an extra-delicious smoothie that you really like. Have a few celery sticks, carrots, or an apple. Have a handful of raw nuts or seeds—but only a handful because although they are healthy, too many can be fattening. Drink a refreshing cup of tea. For the first few days, this will really help to curb your hunger. Look forward to Day 5, then to Day 7, and then to Day 10. Your amazing weight loss results and feelings of high energy will begin to outweigh the longing to eat those less-than-optimal but tempting foods. Rest up and stick with it. You can do this and you will be amazed at the results even after just a few days. Picture yourself telling your story. Go for a walk. Engage in something you thoroughly enjoy doing.

What if my bowels are not moving?

Your bowels should move one to three times per day and never less than once a day. It is absolutely imperative that your bowels move toxins out of your system while cleansing.

If you haven't had a bowel movement in over twenty-four hours, there are two methods to get your bowels moving. Method 1: Use the saltwater flush, which involves drinking uniodized sea salt with water. To tolerate the taste, you can drink two teaspoons of sea salt in eight ounces of water to make it go down and then follow immediately with three more eight-ounce glasses of water. Do this first thing in the morning while you have an empty stomach, and you will have several bowel movements with thirty minutes to an hour. Method 2: One product that really works wonders at getting at the old fecal matter in your colon is Mag07, which I highly recommend. Take three to four pills at bedtime and you can look forward to a heavy bowel movement by morning.

Why are my bowel movements green?

Please don't freak out! It's completely normal and harmless. What you see is chlorophyll (what makes plants green), and it's a good thing. Over time, as your body adjusts to more greens in your diet, your bowel movements will return to their normal brown color.

Can I drink coffee while on the cleanse?

The cleanse is a time to give your body a rest. Coffee containing caffeine gives your adrenal glands a rush, and it is important to take a break from this. Coffee is also acidic. As you cleanse, you are bringing your pH into a more alkaline state, which is imperative for good health. Coffee will interrupt the process of bringing your body into an alkaline state. It is also an irritant to the intestines. Take a break from it for now. If you need to, have a cup of green tea instead. But this also contains caffeine. Going without any caffeinated beverage is best.

For serious coffee drinkers, the hardest part may be giving up coffee. Here's a tip: On the first two days of the cleanse, try half decaf/half regular coffee. For the next two days, try all decaf coffee. After that, try no coffee for the remainder of the cleanse. This will help you gradually ease off coffee so you won't get such strong detox headaches. Additionally, there is an herbal, caffeine-free coffee made by Teeccino that is delicious! And feel free to drink plenty of the herbal teas.

Consider slowly weaning yourself off coffee during the week before you begin the cleanse. You may experience a headache or even achiness during the first few days if you are a regular coffee drinker. Again, this is your body's cleansing reaction. It is very normal to feel less than optimal during the first few days. Consider this a sign that the cleanse is working.

Can I use agave or honey instead of stevia in the smoothies?

Agave is okay in moderation, but if you're interested in weight loss, stevia is the number-one sweetener. The way to think about sweeteners is how much they cause insulin spikes because that determines how much they will cause fat storage in the body. Foods are given glycemic index (GI) ratings according to how much they cause insulin spikes. Stevia is a 0 (which is ideal). Agave is a 20. Honey is about a 30. Brown sugar/raw sugar is a 65. And white refined sugar is an 80. So that gives you some perspective. I have four friends who all use different brands of stevia, and none of us like the others' stevia because they all taste different. If you think you don't like stevia, perhaps just try another brand.

Is the cleanse safe?

It is important to consult with your doctor prior to starting this cleanse. It is unlikely that any damage will be caused by consuming only fruits and vegetables for a period of two weeks or less. Not only is it safe to eat large amounts of plant foods, it may well add years to your life. Blended fruits and vegetables are very cleansing, so there is a possibility that you may experience a reaction as your body cleanses. The more toxic buildup that exists in your system, the more chance you will have of this occurring.

Where can I learn more about green smoothies and get more recipes?

This book contains over 100 green smoothie recipes that are geared toward various health and beauty goals. My favorite books and websites on green smoothies are listed below:

- *Green Smoothie Revolution* by Victoria Boutenko
- Website: www.SimpleGreenSmoothies.com
- Website: www.GreenThickies.com

CHAPTER NINE

Testimonials

Here are just a few of the testimonials from those who did the 10-Day Green Smoothie Cleanse.

"I completed my 10 days yesterday. I lost a total of 15 pounds Woooo-hoooo!! This detox has been such a blessing. JJ Smith, thank you so much for sharing this life-altering plan with us. I learned so much about my body and the importance of clean eating in this short time period. I'm looking forward to a new, healthy life and a positive journey towards my goal weight."

— Nicole F.

"DAY 10!!!! Feeling super excited at how far I've come!!!! I've lost 14 pounds!!!! It's amazing, and I definitely intend to do this again! THANKS, JJ! I'm taking control of my life again and it feels AWESOME!!"

— Mya B.

"I completed Day 10 yesterday and I'm happy to report that I lost a total of (drum roll, please) 13.8 pounds!! Thank you, Jesus! I feel great and am so thankful for JJ Smith and crew for keeping us informed, encouraged, and equipped for this challenge! Just the jumpstart I needed, but more importantly, it opened my eyes to how great natural, raw foods can make me feel. I'm not gonna lie, I started as a skeptic and definitely wasn't expecting to actually feel any different, but I've been converted. Green food = energy, and I'm definitely going to keep going and switch over to the modified version. God bless you all and take care of your temples, ladies!"

— *Felicia B.*

"This is Day 10 for me, and I have lost a total of 15 pounds...I am ecstatic!!!! I must admit, the first three days were quite a challenge for me, but each day thereafter did start to become a lot easier. I'm so proud of me!"

— *Ethel W.*

"Drum roll, please!!!! Day 10 completed and I am down 12 lbs.!!!! What a way to start 2014!!!! Thanks so much, JJ! God Bless you for sharing!! May He continue to enlarge your territory!! We serve an AWESOME God!!"

— *Angela L.*

"Guess what day it is? Day 10, baby!!! I'm here... Boy, I didn't think I was gonna make it, but I kept saying mind/matter you got this. Perseverance...I finished the 10-Day Green Smoothie Cleanse. This was a challenge for me, and it was all mental because I thought I couldn't function without meat. Boy, I feel so much better physically and mentally. I finished the cleanse with a total weight loss of (drum roll, please) 18.4 pounds. I would like to thank JJ Smith for sharing this plan with us. You are a blessing!!"

— Felicia E.

"Day 10 and I must say this have been a great start of a wonderful year. I have lost a total of 14 pounds and 3 inches off my waist. I have great energy and my mind is more clear. I love the energy that I have. I have gotten a lot done. And this will be a forever life change for me. I have been following JJ Smith and am forever grateful for her generous love for others' health and wellness. She is a Rawstar."

—Chantel R.

"Day 10 for me and I am very happy with my results...20 pounds lost. At 55 years old, if I can do it, you can too. I will continue to encourage everyone and thanks again JJ!"

—Freda H.

"Yesterday was Day 10 for me, and I wanted to wait until this morning to weigh myself, and my total weight loss is — drum roll, please — 13 lbs. I will keep this up doing the modified version. I can't wait to go to the doctor's at the end of the month; he's going to be pleased with my weight loss."

—Shelly B.

"Whoo-hoo! Finally, Day 10! I stepped on the scale this morning with my eyes closed, LOL! I'm down 14.5 lbs., from 198 to 183.5. The challenge was HARD but the outcome is AWESOME! And yes, I did have my moments where I ate something to get rid of the headache, but I kept going. In addition, on Day 9 I had a colonics done, which I think really helped!!!"

—*Chablis F.*

"It's Day 11. I am so excited!!! The report is in, and I am down 12.6 lbs.!! YAY!! Thanks, everyone, for the support, and especially you, JJ Smith. The 10-Day Green Smoothie is ROCKIN'. My journey isn't over. I start modified today and am starting out with tea then smoothie and a SALAD for lunch. BTW, my blood pressure has dropped, and I have more energy. YES!!

—*Shonda R.*

"DAY #10, say what? Day #10... I can hardly believe that I have not had any solid food besides apples and boiled eggs (if you considered that solid food??) for 10 whole days and I wasn't sick or in a coma!! LOL! (I Love FOOD). I feel great and I am so proud of myself for staying the course and losing a grand total of 15.8 pounds!!!!!!! I didn't measure myself, so I don't know how many inches, but my clothes tell the story and I feel TERRIFIC!! I must give a big shout out to JJ Smith for her introduction to the green life and a jumpstart to my healthy life. Stay blessed and thank you!"

—*Arlisa B.*

"It's Day 11 and I'm happy to report I'm down 18 lbs.! Wow! Not even to mention my cravings for junk are almost nonexistent. This is so easy compared to other lifestyle changes and by far has given me the best results. Thanks, JJ Smith...you're a beast (in the best way possible), LOL."

—*Gabrielle C.*

"This is Day 11 for me which means...weigh in. (Drum roll, please). I lost 12 lbs. and 8 inches. I feel so good and blessed all over. I can do flips with all the energy I have. I feel and look so healthy. I thank God for this opportunity!"

—*Mia M.*

"It's Day 10 for me, and I'm down 12 pounds! I tried...I did...I saw, I experienced. This is a miracle getting me not to take a sip of coffee for a day, much less 10 days. I am down 12 pounds lighter. Even my five year old said, 'Mommy, you have changed.' Thank you, JJ! I will continue until I achieve my weight goal and get my swag back!"

—*Annette A.*

"I went to the doctor's yesterday because of a knee injury incurred when I took a fall at work. However, the good news is I lost 10 lbs. I was 247 in November, now I am 237, and my blood sugar, which is usually out of control ranging anywhere from 250 to 400, was 78. My doctor was so pleased, as was I. He wants me to stay on the modified cleanse; he agreed that it is helping me a great deal. Now I have to say I really love my smoothies, and while I have to stay with really one kind because of the diabetes, I enjoy them. Well, I will keep you posted."

—*Renee D.*

"10-Day Green Smoothie Cleanse officially finished. Down 14 lbs. Started 10 days ago at 222. Today's weight 208. God bless JJ Smith for sharing this amazing gift with us."

—Ruth C.

"I am excited to say that I ended day 10 yesterday with a new attitude. My energy level is finally up and I'm actually sleeping and resting better. I am craving a big salad, LOL! I am down 15 pounds Woohoo!!!!!! This is just the beginning. I am feeling excited!"

—Lina C.

"Morning of Day 11 and down 13.6 lbs!!! This cleanse has been very life-changing for me. I now have more energy than I ever had, and my skin is glowing. I never had the 'slept like a baby' moment that most had on here, but I am no longer feeling sluggish when I wake up even after four or five hours of sleep (a norm for me)."

—Demetria M.

"Praise the Lord, I have completed my 10 days. I am happy to report 14 pounds down. It doesn't stop here. I will continue with my weight loss journey and a more healthy lifestyle."

—Geraldine C.

"I completed my 10 days yesterday, and I am down 13 lbs. and lost a total of 3 1/2 inches! I want to first thank God for giving me the will and determination to complete this GS cleanse. Once I started, I was determined to finish. My family was very supportive throughout, and I am grateful for that. A big, big thank you goes out to JJ Smith for the info that changed my life forever! I don't feel sluggish anymore like I used to before I started this cleanse, and my health has improved! I will continue to eat healthier from now on. Thank you all for your support!"

—*Tracey W.*

"I want you to know that I lost 12.5 lbs. by Day 6, including 2 inches from my hips and 2 inches from my waist...I'll let you know how much I lost by Day 10. Thanks for introducing me to this cleansing method. I'm sharing it with others."

—*Donna. J.*

"Completed Day 10 and my body responded with 17 lbs.! Thanks, JJ Smith. This group rocks...you are a blessing!"

—*Michelle G.*

"What day is it? What day is it? It's not Wednesday but Day 10 for me!! I did it! JJ, you are truly an angel sent by God, and I thank you for not being selfish with your knowledge and sharing it with me and everyone who desires to be healthy! I want to encourage those who are at the beginning phase of the 10-Day Cleanse: Though no one can go back and make a brand new start, anyone can start from now and make a brand new ending! Oh, I forgot to mention...drum roll, please...I lost a total of 13.2 pounds!! Stay green and stay healthy!"

—*Brenda W.*

"Yesterday was Day 10 of my Green Smoothie Cleanse, and let me just say it was NOT easy but I did it! Glad to report my weight loss of 13 pounds!!!!! I started off at 187 and today I am 174! Thank you, JJ Smith, for the invite and sharing how to be a healthier ME!"

—*Victoria G.*

"Day 10 for me and I'm down 13 pounds. I'm so happy and I feel awesome. I'm gonna continue with the modified version to include the light, healthy meals."

—*Natasha M.*

"Day 10 is like Christmas morning. Couldn't wait to see how much I lost. Just like the good nutritionist said, you can expect to lose nine to fourteen pounds. I did. I am so excited to report on Day 10 I am 13 lbs. smaller, happier, energized, mentally clear, and not to mention caffeine free. I was the queen of java but not anymore. My prayer is that God grant me the strength to keep it up and to lead me not into temptation. I feel like I can keep going on, though. Thank you for your support."

—*Liz P.*

"You are going to love the way this cleanse changes you. I feel great. I have a lot of energy. I'm down 9 lbs. I'm able to go to the bathroom without using supplements, as I've always been constipated. I have continued to cook dinner for him every night, which consisted of T-bone steak, fried chicken, fried fish, mashed potatoes, French fries, bread, and you name it. I don't understand this cleanse, and if I hadn't done it myself I would've thought everyone was lying. It's a mystery but a good mystery. I've never been able to complete any diet. JJ Smith did an amazing job putting this together. I'd like to take this time to thank her for her giving heart. I'm a new me...I plan to do the modified version after my tenth day."

—*Carla S.*

"Holy smokes!! Day 3 for me today, sticking to what is suggested in the book, and I am down 9 pounds!! Yes, 9! I said 9! WOW!! Feeling great!"

—*Olga T.*

"Walked past the mirror and caught a side glimpse of myself. My stomach is GONE!! I know it was there 2 weeks ago! LOL! I cried. Then I danced...and I'm dancing and typing this stat RIGHT NOW!!!! YEEEEEEESSSSS!!!!!!"

—*Natasha W.*

"I completed the 10-Day Detox!! My accomplishment: 9.5 lbs. lost and a total of 7.5 inches smaller. Now Day 1 of modified detox and exercise!!"

—*Nichole W.*

"Yesterday I completed my 10 days!! Down 12 lbs. and lost 12 inches and feeling great! Went to work with smoothie in hand. Had a salad for lunch and have a new appreciation for eating healthy; at lunch literally was mean mugging the greasy option, LOL! Thanks, JJ."

—*Denise B.*

"Day 11 and drum roll...12 pounds down for me and 16 pounds down for the husband, yahhhhh!!!!!!! Now we will continue with the modified version and eating smarter."

—*Carla D.*

"Day 5 and I feel great! Yesterday was a bit of a challenge for me. I've lost 10 pounds as of this morning. I'm totally stoked by this. So as I approach Day 6, I'm beginning to see the light at the end of the tunnel. I know I will finish this cleanse with a bang!"

—*Lalita W.*

"Well, today is my 10th day and I made it! To think that 10 days ago I was worried about finishing. Thank you so much for introducing me to this lifestyle change. I will definitely keep green smoothies in my lifestyle change and as a part of my healthy life. I don't ache when I walk now, I don't have to take painkillers to not be in pain all day, and I get out of bed in the morning with no problem. Loving the new me. I'm even checking out gyms and personal trainers to keep this going. And yes, I lost 11.4 pounds this week."

—*Tonya A.*

"Day 9!! Down 13 pounds, feel great!! I could kick myself for not taking my measurements. Anyway, I'm getting proper rest and it feels good. But I'm shooting for 15 lbs. by the morning of Day 11. LET'S GO!!"

—*Nakia B.*

"This cleanse is simply amazing. This is my Day 6 and I am down 12 pounds. Hopefully I can get off blood pressure meds sooner than later."

—*Jessica L.*

"My husband and I successfully completed Day 10 yesterday!!!! YAYYYY, it was awesome. I lost 12 pounds and my husband lost 10. We enjoyed it so much we've decided to make green smoothies a regular part of our day. I just finished making two pitchers of smoothies for us for tomorrow. Thank you again, JJ Smith."

—*Lisa B.*

"Today is Day 10 for me! I SO proudly announce that I've conquered the 'first round' of any green smoothie cleanse! I visited my team of physicians this afternoon, and they all high-five'd me on my success of losing a whopping 12.5 pounds!! Cheers to us—living with healthier, stronger bodies in 2014!"

—*Darlene B.*

"I AM super fantastic on this here day, 10 pounds lighter, several inches slimmer all over, more limber and flexible, better balanced, with better concentration, vibrant and glowing, energetic, enjoying a flourishing spirit, empowered! Less inflammation and ready to take on 10 more if needed. Dealing daily with chronic fibromyalgia symptoms is not easy and very mental at times, but I'm back in the ring checking in as a heavy weight! Seeking to win the title of a champion! From this achievement and experience, I boldly embrace not just what I learned but what I am becoming! A BETTER ME—THE ME THAT I WAS MEANT TO BE!"

—*Edith B.*

"Yesterday I successfully completed the cleanse. I didn't cheat, no snacks, no stevia, and some days protein powder. I worked out occasionally, LOL. In spite of me not working out like I know I should have, I'm proud of the discipline I gave to this cleanse. I lost a total of 10 pounds, which includes 3 inches off my waist and 2 inches off my hips. I will continue with the modified version until I reach my ultimate goal. I feel vibrant, energized, and my insides feel CLEAN!!!"

—*Davina P.*

"Hey, JJ, my daughter and I completed our 10-Day yesterday, and I'm proud to say that we are both down 12 pounds. Thank you so much for everything. It was the best thing for us to get back in shape and get healthy."

—*Aneesh B.*

"I am feeling good. I have successively completed my 10-Day detox, and I am 11.2 lbs. down!"

—*Victoria C.*

"It's Day 11 and the start of the modified cleanse. I've lost a total of 10 pounds and 2 inches each off of my waist (down at least one dress size), hips, thighs, and chest. I am 5 pounds from my goal weight! I am so happy with the results; now the real work begins in maintaining. Healthy eating is definitely a lifestyle change."

—*Tavia M.*

"Well, folks, it's graduation day today; it is Day 10 for me. I am committing to doing this modified version of 2 smoothies a day until who knows; right now I'm excited and motivated to keep going. I'm 10 pounds down and two sizes down."

—Deborah C.

"I hopped on the scale because my 13-year-old son told me I kind of look different in my stomach area and…drum roll…total of 11 pounds gone forever in 6 days. Woo-hoo!"

—Shatoria A.

"Day 9 for me. I have my two smoothies and snacks in tow and ready for my day. I avoided the scale this morning so I can get a grand total tomorrow. I am already down 14.6 pounds on Day 8, so excited to see tomorrow's total loss. Have a great green day all and stay encouraged—we can do this!"

—Arlisa B.

"Ok, I had to share this excitement…I've been having serious challenges with my high blood pressure, which they call malignant high blood pressure stage 2, and was still not able to control it while under medication. It is heredity, which runs in my family, and the scare I got last month was when the doctor told me, literally, I was a walking time bomb waiting to happen with a severe heart attack, aneurism, or stroke. I have to monitor my readings every day/record my results and give them to my doctor. My pressure was at the over 200 mark over 100, my pulse was even high, past 100.

I would have pain in my head, my eyes, and not to name many others symptoms. It was indeed scary, and to think I am a one year and a half cancer survivor, which when dealing with that was scary, I must admit in itself. So I say all this because today when I took my blood pressure before I had my morning smoothie and meds this morning, to God be the glory, it was 128/89 and my pulse was 74. The last 4 days have been extremely low. I knew I had to make life changes especially with what I have gone through, and I did it before with JJ Smith's help (with her book and guidance), and I knew I could do it again. I owe it to God, my faith, and support system. Much gratitude to JJ!!!! So eating healthy can alter and change many things."

—Stacie J.

"I just finished Day 10 of my cleanse, and I am happy to report that I LOST 11 pounds and that 'I FEEL GOOD' (in my JAMES BROWN voice). I too will be continuing the cleanse, however, with the MODIFIED plan. I want to THANK YOU, JJ Smith, for introducing me to LIVING A HEALTHIER LIFESTYLE!!"

—Renee T.

"On Day 10, and I'm down 10 pounds and feeling great. It has been a wonderful journey that I plan to continue on for a better, healthy life. Congrats to all of you guys. Keep it going!!!!"

—Samantha G.

"Day 9 and I'm feeling fine!!!!! Day 10 tomorrow and I'm gonna party hardy....why?...because I completed what I started, not to mention down 9.8 lbs. off the modified version. If you have fallen off, get back on. Come on and get healthy, you can do it, or still going strong—keep up the awesome work?!"

—*Tiffany D.*

"I'm on Day 10 today and I feel great. Ready to move forward eating healthy as a lifestyle :) I lost 9 lbs. and 4 inches between my bust, hips, and waist. I didn't work out after the 2nd day, and I know I ate more nuts than I should have. I actually cheated on the 3rd night—a bunch of pinches of cheese pizza. I truly believe you started a movement that is needed for our people, and I pray God blesses you because I know you didn't have to do this. Now that's what I call integrity! Keep doing what you're doing, my sister—people are watching."

—*Tunisia S.*

"Day 7 and down 10 pounds!!!!! This is the best thing I could have ever done for myself. I'm proud I stayed on track and didn't cheat. I noticed my face looks brighter and clearer. I'm going to exercise this morning!"

—*Natasha M.*

"I lost 16 inches!!! I'm so freakin' excited!!!!

—*Cee M.*

"I am on Day 6 and I am down 9 pounds. I think I can make it now. I love the results and plan to continue this."

—*Beverly A.*

"I'm excited. It's Day 4 for me. I decided to get on the scale this morning and discovered 10 lbs. gone. Yay me!"

—*Stephanie S.*

"Getting ready to start my Day 3, and I know JJ Smith said don't focus really on the weight loss, but I could not help myself. I weighed myself this morning to find out I have lost pounds...Yes, 8 whole pounds. Feeling good and refreshed, ready to work it!"

—*Janice D.*

CHAPTER TEN

Success Stories

Here are a few success stories from people who completed the 10-Day Green Smoothie Cleanse.

"This 10 day green smoothie cleanse has been amazing!"

"I'm feeling more energetic, my eyes are clear, lower back pain has decreased, and I'm in an overall great mood. It has been awesome, I can literally feel my body go into happy mode when I have a smoothie. It just says ahhhhhhhhhh!!! Today is day 10. I have lost 13 pounds as of yesterday. I wasn't really clocking the scale, but I have noticed the belly fat melting away. I don't feel bloated. My mood is steady. I was a bit cranky the first day or so, but it quickly went away. This cleanse has most definitely helped me continue to reach my fitness goals and I look forward to this ongoing lifestyle change. Thanks to JJ Smith for her vision of health for people."

—*Wilson G.*

"I lost 14 pounds in 10 days and have clarity and more focus!"

"10-Day Green Smoothie should be renamed to more energy, proper sleep, and a healthier you. Because that's exactly what I feel. My insomnia is going. I have more energy than my mind can keep up with. I'm more conscious when I pick up something to purchase to eat. I dropped 14 pounds, which is a blessing for me. I have clarity and I'm more focused. Go figure! Change your diet, change your life. This is not just a 10-day cleanse, this is a life-changing cleansing. For all of you that struggle in the beginning of the cleanse, your body and your mind will thank you for it later. The headaches will subdue, and your skin will be radiant. And your energy level will sky rocket. Thanks for this life-changing experience."

—Chantel R.

"I lost 15 pounds in 10 days and have a renewed life!"

"You see, I have been abusing food for the last seven or eight years, and my body definitely suffered as a result. I stepped on the scale New Year's Eve, and I was at my heaviest weight in my entire life. On January 1, 2014, with much prayer and excitement, I began the 10-Day Green Smoothie Cleanse. I cannot even say it was challenging because I felt more and more awesome with each passing day. So on to the good stuff. Here's what this cleanse did for my body:

- I lost a total of 15 pounds in 10 days.
- My energy level has soared.

- My body aches and pains have disappeared.
- I realized I don't need that cup of coffee in the morning to start my day. I'm actually energized.
- The bottom of my feet ached for months so badly that I thought I had plantar fasciitis. Since I've done the cleanse, the pain is there but very minimal.
- I had very sensitive areas in my mouth. That pain is completely gone.
- My hair, which seemed so brittle for years, actually felt strong and healthy. I could comb through it with little to no breakage (a first in years).
- My fingernails are rock hard.
- When I started the cleanse, I felt a sinus infection coming on. My body self-cured the infection without antibiotics (another first for me).
- Last but not least, I feel motivated, inspired, and accomplished.

Stumbling upon this cleanse has been more than a blessing. It gave me renewed life. JJ, thank you so much for sharing your knowledge freely with so many people."

—*Nicole F.*

"My weight today is 23 pounds less than when I began this journey 12 days ago!"

"Have you ever had a time in your life when you couldn't see a reason to get up and out? I have. It wasn't because of illness or depression, it was mainly because I didn't have the motivation. Yes, I'm a mother, wife, business owner, house keeper, nurse...the list goes on and on. There have been piles and piles of stress dropped on me, some of which I have placed on myself needlessly. With this stress came poor time management.

I tried different diet and exercise plans to change the weight, and I would be successful for a while. Then yet another stress would jump on my back and I would put off the plan...for just a little while. I was not able to walk for a long time because my feet and back hurt. I hadn't slept a full night in 16 years. Sleeping was more difficult recently because I would wake up at all hours to the numbness and burning in my hands.

"Fast forward to 2013. I am tired, menopause is setting in, and I try to work out but I am so lethargic. I see doctors who tell me just to lift weights. Really?? I start working out in November and things are okay. On the bike for one to two hours (oh, did I say I was supplementing with caffeine to stay up?) and lifting weights. I cut way down on eating...I know, I know, just to see the scale go down. In eight weeks' time, I had only lost eight pounds. Sadness.

"Then my friend had a post about this green cleanse. Hmm, I thought. This looks interesting. I jumped in. Since that first smoothie, and I do mean first, I have felt energized. I have slept nearly the whole night. I don't have the numbing, burning in my hands, and I even park great distances away to walk into buildings. Let the other folks have the 'good' spots. My weight today is 23 pounds less than when I began this journey 12 days ago.

Darn, I can pull my pants off without unzipping them! LOL, talk about joy! I can take the stairs with greater ease and have played not only with my young son, but with our dog. I'm able to work out in the morning, have a full day at work, cook, clean and study without saying that dreaded 'I'm so tired' like I used to. It seemed to be the only excuse I had in my vocabulary. But no more. This is all because of the blessed and highly favored JJ Smith and her remarkable 10-Day Green Smoothie Cleanse."

—Maria W.

"He lost 21 pounds and his blood pressure is now perfect!"

"I have the best father in the WORLD! When I said to him that he needed to do a detox, he did not question me. He trusted what I was telling him. My father has battled high blood pressure for as long as I can remember. Well, I have been on a health-learning journey for about two years now where I have learned amazing things about health. I have read several of JJ's books, documentaries, etc. Halfway through the cleanse, I asked my dad if he felt any different. He said that he had more energy and that he was now able to walk up stairs without stopping to rest. Well, you cannot even understand the joy I felt. I felt accomplished. I felt that as long as my dad is good, I am most certainly good.

My dad and I completed the cleanse this past Tuesday. Woo-hoo!!! This Thursday he went to the doctor for his scheduled doctor's appointment and, drum roll, he had lost 21 pounds. Yes, 21 pounds. The doctor had been after him to lose weight for months. I'm not finished yet – his blood pressure was PERFECT!!! The doctor and the nurse asked him what was he doing, and JJ, he gave all the credit to me, but I give the credit to YOU and HIM. This man did not complain or anything; he did whatever I said he needed to do, which was what you said to do. He and I are continuing on this health journey with the green smoothies. JJ, again, thank you so very much for sharing your knowledge, caring, and your support!

—*Tara L.*

"I am down 17 pounds and thinking clearer, feeling great and sleeping like never before!"

Today is day 11 and still going strong!! I must admit I didn't think that I would finish after looking at all this green stuff (vegetables that is), but through a lot of prayer and soul searching I completed the cleanse on yesterday. I am thinking I clearer, feeling great, sleeping like never before and the energy I have now reminds me of my years gone by. I will not be going back to the way of eating like before. For the better news for me, I am down 17 pounds, pants falling down, shirts to loose, blood pressure is now at 113/67, 2 inches off waist and 3 inches off my stomach. I would like to say a big thanks to JJ Smith for your time and honesty about what will happen during this cleanse. You are helping to save many if we just be honest with ourselves and realize we can't do this alone. I am on a new journey to healthy green living?."

—*Mike B.*

"I'm more energized, alert, no digestive problems, with clearer skin and eyes."

"Well, I must admit I was going through some disappointment of putting on 10 pounds after turning 50 in August. When I began this journey 10 days ago, I was so excited. So as I completed Day 10, I've noticed these changes: I'm more energized, alert, no digestive problems, clearer skin and eyes, not sleepy at work after lunch to name a few celebrations.

As I ended my Day 10 yesterday, I will continue with the modified plan of replacing 2 meals with a green smoothie. I still have at least 15 more pounds that I would like to lose to remain healthy. I'm choosing to LIVE and not DIE. I guess you want to know what my measurements and weight results were. Here they are:

- Weight — 10 lbs. lighter
- Bust — 1 inch
- Waist — 2 inches
- Hips — 3 inches
- Thighs — 2 inches left, 1 inch right

"Thanks, Green Team, and continue to press toward the mark of the high calling, which is a better health for us all."

—*Wendy M.*

"My 10-Day Smoothie Cleanse Detox Experience."

1. I controlled my snack portions and prepped them for the first time EVER!

2. Lost 5 inches from my waist
3. Slept better and had more energy
4. My skin is clearer
6. I learned to substitute my soda cravings with fresh red grapefruit and stevia
7. I invested in whole foods and changed my perspective on the costs
8. Committed to myself and saw this plan all the way through
9. Gained clarity that food should not be a comforting escape but instead an energy source
10. Ran faster during my workouts
11. FINALLY...I lost 14 pounds and counting!!

"Thanks to JJ Smith for your support! I plan to continue with the modified version and later jump on board for another 10 days next month! God Bless You!"

—*Chiara M.*

"This is just what I needed to jump-start me into action!"

"12 ? cans of soda, 29.4 glasses of wine, 36 sticks of butter, 42 chicken wings, 98 chocolate bars. Pick your poison, but THAT is what is lost in the last 10 days! Not only that, I have lost much much more! Oh, yeah, the restless nights are gone, too. I am sleeping like a baby and falling asleep without issue! The mini black purses I carried under my eyes...well, not completely gone but very much diminished to the point I can claim they are gone! Dry, not-so-supple skin...also gone! Replaced with touch-me-now, no-makeup-required skin; I know it's not healthy, but I cannot stop touching my face! Belly, yup, gone too! Also gone is that uncomfortable feeling associated with clothes, walking, breathing…you name it! GONE!

"I still have a ways to go, but this is just what I needed to jump-start me into action! I began at 165.4 pounds and am down to 156.2. I am glad I saw this through, as I am now motivated to continue. My cravings for junk have died and have been replaced with cravings for health, wellness, and happiness. Next up…DEM Plan for maintenance! Thanks again to JJ for another great resource! I purchased the book (*Lose Weight Without Dieting or Working Out*) over a year ago, but I now have the mental clarity and motivation to see it through! My reward: a long overdue mani/pedi and a fabulous me! Good luck to those just starting and for those new to the program. See it through—you will be amazed at yourself and the results!"

—*Latrisse P.*

"I am 9 pounds lighter and, most importantly, have a new relationship with food!"

"So today was my Day 10, and I must say I feel so much better than I did 11 days ago. Since September, I have been on and off a diet. But I realized diets don't work, and with this I realize it has to be an entire lifestyle change for me to yield and keep the results that I want. So with that said, I am 9 pounds lighter and, most importantly, I have a new perspective on my relationship with food in general. I want to thank EVERYONE for their support. I will keep everyone posted."

—*Star S.*

"Completing this cleanse revealed that I AM in control of what I put in my body!"

"I am ECSTATIC to report that I successfully completed the cleanse and I still feel AMAZING! To be completely honest, I didn't approach the cleanse with a positive attitude at all! I didn't believe I could do it. I didn't believe it would change me. My excuses have always been, 'Nothing else has worked so why would this be any different?' and 'I'm fighting my genetic makeup...everyone in my family has weight issues.'

I don't know how much weight I've lost because I didn't step on the scale before the cleanse, mainly because fear kept me from facing the truth. The truth about my poor eating habits and lack of discipline. Completing this cleanse revealed that I AM in control of what I put in my body, I CAN fight urges, I AM disciplined, and I CAN practice healthy eating habits. I actually believe it!!!"

—Karen W.

"I have experienced great results! No more muffin top!"

"I completed my 10th Day yesterday! I have experienced great results! No more muffin top! I can now fit my size 4 clothing, which is a good thing since I no longer have anything larger than that in my closet to wear! A special thank you to JJ Smith; it all started with me purchasing her book How to *Lose Weight without Dieting or Working Out*. The methods in that book worked and helped me achieve my goal size 4, so I knew when she put this together it would work as well.

"The next thing I did was change my mindset. You must

decide in your mind that it's something you need to do. I also visualized the end result—for some it might be a Beyoncé body. For me it was seeing myself wearing a size 4! If you are new or not, stay plugged into it during your detox journey!"

—Nicole H.

CHAPTER ELEVEN

Conclusion

I want to say congrats on taking this amazing first step to take back control of your weight and health. If you are reading this, you've already done the hard part, and that's to make the decision to lose weight and get healthy. You are on your way. This is a journey that will change your life—it's not a diet but a lifestyle!

Remember that you have the power to change your life, and now with the information in this book, you have the tools to turn your dreams into reality. Every day is the beginning of the rest of your life. You are in control of what happens today. Start dreaming about a healthy, beautiful body and watch it become reality. You have power over your body and your life, so live it with passion because you only get one!

In closing, I want to leave you with my *10 Commandments for Looking Young and Feeling Great*, which I always share at the end of my teleseminars.

1. ***Thou shalt love thyself.*** Self-love is essential to survival. There is no successful, authentic relationship with others without self-love. We cannot water the

land from a dry well. Self-love is not selfish or self-indulgent. We have to take care of our needs first so we can give to others from abundance.

2. *Thou shalt take responsibility for thine own health and well-being.* If you want to be healthy, have more energy, and feel great, you must take the time to learn what is involved and apply it to your own life. You have to watch what goes into your mouth, how much exercise and physical activity you get, and what thoughts you're thinking throughout the day.

3. *Thou shalt sleep.* Sleep and rest is the body's way of recharging the system. Sleep is the easiest yet most underrated activity for healing the body. Lack of sleep definitely saps your glow and instantly ages you, giving you puffy red eyes with dark circles under them.

4. *Thou shalt detoxify and cleanse the body*. Detoxifying the body means ridding the body of poisons and toxins so that you can speed up weight loss and restore great health. A clean body is a beautiful body!

5. *Thou shalt remember that a healthy body is a sexy body.* Real women's bodies look beautiful! It's about getting healthy and having style and confidence and wearing clothes that match your body type.

6. *Thou shalt eat healthy, natural, whole foods.* Healthy eating can turn back the hands of time and return the body to a more youthful state. When you eat natural foods, you simply look and feel better. You keep the body clean at the cellular level and look radiant despite your age. Eating healthy should be part of your "beauty regimen."

7. ***Thou shalt embrace healthy aging.*** The goal is not to stop the aging process but to embrace it. Healthy aging is staying healthy as you age, which is looking and feeling great despite your age.

8. ***Thou shalt commit to a lifestyle change.*** Losing weight permanently requires a commitment to changes...in your thinking, your lifestyle, your mindset. It requires gaining knowledge and making permanent changes in your life for the better!

9. ***Thou shalt embrace the journey.*** This is a journey that will change your life; it's not a diet but a lifestyle! Be kind and supportive to yourself. Learn to applaud yourself for the smallest accomplishment. And when you slip up sometimes, know that it is okay; it is called being human.

10. ***Thou shalt live, love, and laugh.*** Laughter is still good for the soul. Live your life with passion! Never give up on your dreams! And most importantly... love! Remember that love never fails!

Now that you have experienced the power of the 10-Day Green Smoothie Cleanse, be sure to share your success story with others and help them to reclaim their health and vitality.

Over 100 Green Smoothie Recipes for Different Goals

*I*n chapter 2, I listed the most popular greens, as well as the milder- and stronger-tasting greens, that you can choose for the recipes below. The typical amount of greens you should use for each recipe is about two handfuls. If you want to make the green smoothie sweeter, feel free to add stevia to your preferred taste.

Blending instructions: Place the leafy greens and whatever liquids are called for (or ice) into the blender and blend until the mixture is a juice-like consistency. Stop the blender and add the remaining ingredients. Blend until creamy.

Anti-Aging

Peach Banana Greens

2 handfuls greens

2 cups water

1½ cups frozen peaches

1 banana, peeled

2 tablespoons sunflower oil

2 teaspoons spirulina

Berry Coconut

2 handfuls greens

1½ cups coconut water

½ cup frozen blueberries

½ cup frozen raspberries

Watermelon Ginger Greens

2 handfuls greens

½ cup ice

4 cups watermelon chunks

2 tablespoons chia seeds

1 inch fresh ginger, peeled

Banana Nut Greens

2 handfuls greens

1½ cups almond milk

3 bananas, peeled

2 tablespoons chia seeds

Athletic Performance

Berry Protein Greens

2 handfuls greens

2 cups water

1½ cups frozen raspberries

¼ cup frozen blueberries

¼ cup almond butter

¼ cup cacao powder

½ cup plant-based protein powder

Banana Rice Protein

2 cups chopped celery

2 cups ice

⅓ cup cashews

3 bananas, peeled

½ cup plant-based protein powder

1 tablespoon spirulina

Cherry Wheatgrass

2 handfuls greens

1 cup water

1 cup frozen cherries

½ cup fresh wheatgrass juice

½ cup fresh beet juice

¼ cup chia seeds

4 large pitted dates

Berry Seeds

2 handfuls greens

2 cups water

1 cup frozen blueberries

½ cup sunflower seeds

½ cup chia seeds

6 dried figs

2 pitted dates

1 cup cacao powder

Nut Celery Protein

1 handful greens

2 cups water

½ cup macadamia nuts

¼ cup fresh wheatgrass juice

4 large pitted dates

1 cup chopped celery

½ cup plant-based protein powder

Berry Pumpkin Protein

2 handfuls greens

½ cup chopped celery

2 cups water

½ cup pumpkin seeds

¼ cup goji berries

4 pitted dates

½ cup plant-based protein powder

2 tablespoons maca powder

Banana Sunflower Protein

2 handfuls greens

1 cup water

½ cup sunflower seeds

2 pitted dates

2 bananas, peeled

1 cup plant-based protein powder

1 tablespoon ginseng powder

Beauty (Healthy Hair, Skin, and Nails)

Mango Banana

2 handfuls greens

1 cup coconut water

1 banana, peeled

1½ cups frozen mango chunks

Papaya Lemon

1 handful parsley

2 cups water

1 banana, peeled and frozen

1 cup papaya chunks

1 lemon

Orange Spinach

2 cups baby spinach

1 orange, peeled and seeded

1 kiwi, peeled

1 tablespoon apple cider vinegar

1 packet stevia

Banana Pear

2 handfuls greens

1½ cups water

1 banana, peeled and frozen

2 pears

⅓ cup almond butter

Apple Pear

2 handfuls greens

2 stalks celery, chopped

½ cup water

1 pear, seeded

1 large apple

1 banana, peeled and frozen

2 tablespoons fresh lemon juice

Green Berry

2 handfuls greens

½ cup water

½ cup green tea

2 cups mixed berries

1 banana, peeled and frozen

Carrot Apple

2 handfuls greens

3 stalks celery

1 cup water

1 small beet, peeled and diced

1 cup ice

2 carrots

1 apple

½ lemon, seeded, peeled, and sectioned

Cranberry Berry

2 handfuls greens

½ cup ice

½ cup blueberries

½ cup blackberries

½ cup cranberries

1 tablespoon ground chia seeds

Cucumber Strawberry

2 handfuls greens

1 cup water

1 cucumber

1 cup frozen strawberries

4 dried figs

2 tablespoons ground flaxseeds

Bones and Joints

Banana Berry

2 handfuls greens

2 cups water

1 cup frozen blueberries

1 banana, peeled

2 tablespoons ground chia seeds

Banana Nut

2 handfuls greens

1 cup almond milk

2 bananas, peeled and frozen

2 tablespoons cacao

2 tablespoons ground flaxseeds

Orange Avocado

2 handfuls greens

1 cup water

½ cup ice

3 oranges, peeled

½ avocado, peeled and pitted

2 teaspoons spirulina powder

Lemon Zest

2 handfuls greens

1½ cups fresh-squeezed orange juice

1 cup ice

1 lemon, peeled

1 tablespoon MSM powder

Ginger Pear

2 handfuls greens

1 cup almond milk

2 large pears

1 inch fresh ginger, peeled

Constipation

Beet Pears

2 handfuls greens

1½ cups almond milk

2 large pears

¼ cup beets, peeled and diced

Banana Blueberry

2 handfuls greens

1 cup water

1 pear

1 banana, peeled and frozen

1 cup frozen blueberries

Banana Prunes

2 handfuls greens

1½ cups almond milk

2 bananas, peeled and frozen

5 prunes, seeded

1 pear

Orange Mango

2 handfuls greens

1 cup water

1 cup frozen mango chunks

2 oranges, peeled and seeded

Strawberry Kiwi

2 handfuls greens

1 cup water

1½ cup frozen strawberries

2 kiwis (skin on)

2 tablespoons flaxseeds

Detoxification

Lemon Lime

2 handfuls greens

1 large fresh-squeezed orange

½ cup of ice

2 bananas, peeled and frozen

½ lemon, peeled and seeded

½ lime, peeled and seeded

Blackberry Banana

2 handfuls greens

¼ cup water

1 banana, peeled and frozen

½ cup frozen blackberries

1 cup frozen strawberries

1 cup frozen blueberries

Grapefruit Banana

2 handfuls greens

1 cup water

1 banana, peeled and frozen

1 cup frozen strawberries

1 pink grapefruit, peeled and seeded

1 packet stevia

Pear Pineapple

2 handfuls greens

1 cup ice

1 pear, seeded

1 small apple, cored and seeded

2 cups pineapple chunks

Mango Pineapple

2 handfuls greens

1½ cups coconut water

1 cup frozen mango chunks

1 cup pineapple chunks

1 lime, peeled and seeded

Pinch of cayenne pepper

Apple Banana

2 handfuls greens

1 cup ice

2 granny smith apples, cored and seeded

2 small bananas, peeled

Diabetes/Blood Sugar Control

Orange Plum

2 handfuls greens

½ cup ice

2 oranges, peeled

½ cup plums

1 teaspoon cinnamon

2 tablespoons ground flaxseeds

Pear Banana

2 handfuls greens

1 cup almond milk

1 banana, peeled and frozen

1 pear

1 apple, cored and seeded

1 teaspoon cinnamon

Kiwi Almond

2 handfuls greens

1½ cups almond milk

1 banana, peeled and frozen

2 kiwis (skin on)

1 cup frozen strawberries

2 tablespoons ground flaxseeds

Berry Banana

2 handfuls greens

1 cup water

1 banana, peeled and frozen

1½ cups frozen blueberries

2 tablespoons ground flaxseeds

Mango Almond

2 handfuls greens

1½ cups almond milk

½ cup frozen mango chunks

1 cup frozen strawberries

Mango Orange

2 handfuls greens

1 cup water

½ cup frozen mango chunks

½ lemon, peeled and seeded

1 orange, peeled and seeded

2 tablespoons sunflower seeds

Avocado Greens

2 handfuls greens

1 cup ice

1 medium banana, peeled

2 cups frozen strawberries

¼ avocado, peeled

Orange Berry Seeds

2 handfuls greens

1 cup unsweetened almond milk

1 small orange, peeled

½ cup frozen mixed berries

1 teaspoon goji berries, soaked for 10 minutes

1 tablespoon ground flaxseeds

1 scoop of plant-based protein powder

Energy

Strawberry Grape

2 handfuls greens

½ cup water

½ cup red grapes

2 bananas, peeled and frozen

1½ cups frozen strawberries

Minty Pears

2 handfuls greens

½ cup water

2 pears

¼-inch section of fresh ginger, grated

¼ cup chopped fresh mint leaves

Pear Orange

2 handfuls greens

½ cup ice

1 pear, cored and seeded

2 oranges, peeled and seeded

1 tablespoon of ground flaxseeds

Peachy Mango

2 handfuls greens

1 cup water

1½ cups frozen peaches

2 nectarines, peeled, cored, and seeded

1 cup frozen mango chunks

2 plums, cored and seeded

Coconut Berries

2 handfuls greens

1 cup water

2 nectarines, peeled, cored, and seeded

1 banana, peeled and frozen

½ cup goji berries

½ cup shredded coconut

Heart Health

Banana Mango

2 handfuls greens

2 cups water

1 banana, peeled and frozen

½ cup frozen mango chunks

2 teaspoons spirulina

2 tablespoons walnut oil

Banana Almond

2 handfuls greens

1½ cups almond milk

3 bananas, peeled and frozen

½ teaspoon cinnamon

Coconut Berry

2 handfuls greens

1 cup coconut water

1 cup frozen blueberries

¼ cup goji berries

Watermelon Mint

2 handfuls greens

4 cups watermelon

2 tablespoons ground flaxseeds

Sunflower Orange

2 handfuls greens

1 cup water

2 oranges, peeled and seeded

1 cup red grapes

2 tablespoons ground flaxseeds

2 tablespoons sunflower oil

Avocado Apple

2 handfuls greens

1 cup unsweetened apple juice

1 cup ice

2 small apples, cored and seeded

½ avocado, peeled and cored

¼ cup beets, peeled and diced

1 tablespoon cacao powder

Peach Berry

2 handfuls greens

1 cup water

1½ cups frozen peaches

1 cup mixed berries

½ avocado, peeled and cored

Pear Banana

2 handfuls greens

1½ cups almond milk

2 pears

1 banana, peeled and frozen

½ teaspoon vanilla extract

Immune Boosting

Cantaloupe Carrot

2 handfuls greens

½ cup green tea

1 banana, peeled and frozen

1 carrot, chopped

1 cup cantaloupe, peeled, seeded, and chopped

1 packet stevia

Green Strawberry

2 handfuls greens

½ cup green tea

½ cups frozen strawberries

1 banana, peeled and frozen

1 packet stevia

Strawberry Orange

2 handfuls greens

½ cup water

2 cups frozen strawberries

1 large orange, peeled and seeded

1 packet stevia

Mango Blackberry

2 handfuls greens

1 cup water

½ cup frozen blackberries

½ cup frozen raspberries

1 cup frozen mango chunks

1 orange, peeled and seeded

1 packet stevia

Banana Lemon

2 handfuls greens

1 cup ice

1 banana, peeled and frozen

½ cup green grapes

1 lemon, seeded and peeled

1 packet stevia

Kid-Friendly

Orange Apricot

2 handfuls greens

1 cup water

2 oranges, peeled and seeded

6 dried apricots, pitted

1 banana, peeled and frozen

½ cup almonds

¼ cup almond butter

Berry Banana

2 handfuls greens

1 cup water

1 large banana, peeled and frozen

1¼ cups frozen blueberries

¼ cup ground flaxseeds

1 packet stevia

Chocolate Nut

2 handfuls greens

2 cups water

½ cup cashew nuts

½ cup raw cacao powder

6 large pitted dates

1 packet stevia

Chocolate Banana

2 handfuls greens

1½ cups water

2 bananas, peeled and frozen

1 cup hazelnut butter

4 large pitted dates

¼ cup raw cacao powder

Blackberry Almond

1 handful greens

2 cups almond milk

1 banana, peeled and frozen

½ cup frozen blueberries

1 cup frozen blackberries

2 pitted dates

Berry Almond

1 handful greens

1½ cups almond milk

2 teaspoons fresh lemon juice

2 cups frozen mixed berries

¼ cup goji berries

6 large pitted dates

1 packet stevia

Berry Medley

1 handful greens

1½ cups cashew milk

2½ cups frozen mixed berries

4 large pitted dates

2 teaspoons vanilla extract

Mood-Enhancing

Berry Beets

2 handfuls greens

1 cup water

1 banana, peeled and frozen

1½ cups frozen peaches

1 cup frozen blueberries

½ beet, peeled and diced

1 carrot, chopped

Mango Walnut

2 handfuls greens

1½ cups almond milk

1½ cups frozen mango chunks

1 banana, peeled and frozen

1 tablespoon walnut oil

Banana Nectarine

2 handfuls greens

1 cup water

2 bananas, peeled and frozen

1 nectarine, peeled and pitted

1 cup frozen strawberries

3 pitted dates

Berry Medley Banana

2 handfuls greens

1½ cups water

1 banana, peeled and frozen

2 cups frozen mixed berries

2 tablespoons ground flaxseeds

Red Berry Medley

2 handfuls greens

1 cup water

2 small red apples, cored and seeded

1 cup frozen strawberries

Papaya Greens

2 handfuls greens

½ cup ice

1 papaya, peeled and seeded

1¼ cups fresh pineapple chunks

Banana Coconut

2 handfuls greens

½ cup ice

2 bananas, peeled and frozen

1 lime, peeled and seeded

½ cup shredded coconut

¼ cup fresh chopped coconut

1 cup coconut water

½ avocado, peeled and pitted

Avocado Banana

2 handfuls greens

½ cup ice

2 oranges, peeled and seeded

1 banana, peeled and frozen

½ avocado, peeled and pitted

Pear Vanilla

2 handfuls greens

1 cup almond milk

½ cup ice

1 apple

1 banana, peeled and frozen

1 pear

2 tablespoons ground flaxseeds

1 teaspoon vanilla extract

Stress

Pineapple Greens

2 handfuls greens

1 cup water

2 cups pineapple chunks

1 cup frozen peaches

1 banana, peeled and frozen

Grapefruit Banana

2 handfuls greens

1 cup coconut water

1 pink grapefruit, peeled and seeded

2 kiwis

1 banana, peeled and frozen

Pomegranate Berry

2 handfuls greens

½ cup pomegranate juice

1 banana, peeled and frozen

½ cup frozen blueberries

½ cup strawberries

½ cup red grapes

Apple Banana Greens

2 cups water

2 handfuls greens

2 small apples, cored and seeded

2 bananas, peeled and frozen

1 pear, seeded

1 tablespoon ground chia seeds

Weight Loss and Fat Burning

Fat-Burner Smoothie

2 handfuls greens

2 cups cooled green tea

½ can coconut milk

Juice of 1 lemon

¼ cup pitted dates

½ avocado, peeled and pitted

½ pink grapefruit, peeled and seeded

Orange Banana Greens

2 handfuls greens

½ cup water

2 oranges, peeled and seeded

2 bananas, peeled and frozen

Berry Pears

2 handfuls greens

1½ cups almond milk

2 cups frozen mixed berries

2 pears, seeded

Banana Berry Almond

2 handfuls greens

1½ cups almond milk

1 banana, peeled and frozen

1 cup frozen blueberries

½ cup frozen strawberries

Berry Cantaloupe

2 handfuls greens

1 cup water

½ cantaloupe, peeled and seeded

1½ cups frozen strawberries

Cherry Orange

2 handfuls greens

1½ cups almond milk

1 cup cherries, pitted

2 oranges, peeled and seeded

1 tablespoon ground chia seeds

Raspberry Orange

2 handfuls greens

½ cup water

2 oranges, peeled and seeded

2 cups frozen raspberries

Peachy Vanilla

2 handfuls greens

1 cup water

1½ cups frozen peaches

1 cup frozen strawberries

1 teaspoon vanilla extract

Mango Lime

2 handfuls greens

1½ cups water

1 orange, peeled and seeded

½ cup frozen mango chunks

1 lime, peeled and seeded

1 packet stevia

Green Raspberry

2 handfuls greens

1 cup water

1 banana, peeled and frozen

1 cup frozen raspberries

2 tablespoons ground flaxseeds

Chia Pear

2 handfuls greens

1½ cups water

1 banana, peeled and frozen

2 pears

2 tablespoons ground chia seeds

Pineapple Orange Greens

2 handfuls greens

1 cup ice

1 cup pineapple chunks

2 oranges peeled and seeded

Watermelon Greens

2 handfuls greens

1 cup ice

2 cups watermelon

1 teaspoon ground flaxseeds

Grapefruit Pineapple

2 handfuls greens

½ cup coconut water

½ cup ice

1 cup pineapple chunks

1 pink grapefruit

Miscellaneous

The Complete Meal Smoothie

2 handfuls greens

1 cup unsweetened almond milk

½ cup water

1 cup frozen blueberries (or mixed berries)

2 tablespoons low-fat Greek yogurt

1 tablespoon ground flaxseeds

Stevia, to taste

Banana Chia Smoothie

2 handfuls greens

½ cup water or crushed ice

1 banana, peeled and frozen

1 cup raspberries (fresh or frozen)

2 teaspoons chia seeds (soaked for 10 minutes)

Coconut Peach Smoothie

2 handfuls greens

1 cup coconut water

2 cups frozen grapes

2 peaches, pitted

Tropical Spinach Smoothie

2 handfuls greens

2 cups water

1 cup pineapple chunks

1 cup mango chunks

2 bananas, peeled and frozen

Chocolate Cherry Smoothie

2 handfuls greens

2 cups unsweetened almond milk

2 cups cherries, pitted

2 bananas, peeled and frozen

1 teaspoon cinnamon

3 tablespoons cacao powder

Orange Berry Spinach Smoothie

2 handfuls greens

1 cup ice

1 large orange, peeled, seeded, and segmented

½ large banana, cut into chunks

6 large frozen strawberries

⅓ cup plain Greek yogurt

Ginger Green Smoothie

2 handfuls greens

2 cups water

1 banana, cut into chunks

1 orange, peeled and separated into segments

½ apple (your favorite variety), cored, seeded, cut into chunks

½ lemon, peeled, seeded

½-inch piece of fresh ginger, peeled and minced

Coconut Mango Spinach Smoothie

2 handfuls greens

1½ cups water

1 cup frozen coconut milk/coconut water

1 cup frozen mango

1 packet stevia

1 tablespoon hemp protein powder

Blueberry Bliss Smoothie

1 cup spinach

2 cups water

1 cup frozen blueberries

1 banana, peeled

Cherry Smoothie

2 handfuls greens

1 cup coconut milk (or replace with water to reduce the calories)

1 cup almond milk

2 cups cherries

½ cup raisins

1 cup of oats (you will chew them in the smoothie)

Banana Peach Kale Smoothie

2 handfuls greens

1½ cups water

1 cup almond milk

1 cup frozen peaches

1 banana, peeled and frozen

1 cup oats

¼ cup dried apricots (or any other dried fruit)

¼ cup almonds (use ground almonds if you don't have a high-speed blender)

APPENDIX B

Clean, High-Protein Recipes

*I*n chapter 6, I discuss eating clean, high-protein meals to assist with weight loss after the cleanse. Here are a few of my favorite recipes that are clean, healthy, and delicious!

Baked Salmon
in Spicy Lime-Cilantro Dressing

1 pound salmon fillet, skinned

1 chili pepper, seeded and cut into thin strips

⅓ cup fresh limejuice

2 green onions, sliced

1 cup packed fresh cilantro leaves, chopped

1 teaspoon canola oil

½ teaspoon sea salt

1. Preheat oven to 350°F.
2. Combine chili pepper, limejuice, onions, cilantro, oil, and salt in a food processor and purée.
3. Place salmon in a baking dish just large enough to fit fillet. Pour sauce from blender over salmon, turning fish to coat on both sides.
4. Bake, uncovered, until fish is cooked to your liking in center, 20 to 25 minutes depending on thickness of the fish.
5. To serve, slice fillet into pieces and spoon sauce over each portion.

Almond-Crusted Baked Chicken

3 medium chicken breasts

2 egg whites

1 cup almonds

¼ cup parmesan cheese

1 teaspoon thyme

2 teaspoons oregano

1 teaspoon sea salt

1. Preheat oven to 350° F.
2. Place almonds, oregano, parmesan cheese, sea salt, and thyme into a food processor and process until well blended.
3. Place chicken on one plate, egg whites in a shallow bowl, and almond mixture on a second plate.
4. Gently roll each piece of chicken in egg whites, then in the almond mixture, and place on parchment-lined baking sheet.
5. Bake for about 30 minutes.

Scallops with Lemon Sauce

1½ pounds sea scallops, washed and dried

¼ cup fresh parsley leaves

2 tablespoons fresh lemon juice

¼ cup extra-virgin olive oil

1 garlic clove, minced

½ teaspoon sea salt

¼ teaspoon ground pepper

1. Combine the lemon juice, parsley, garlic, sea salt, and pepper in a small bowl.
2. Whisk the olive oil into combined ingredients and set it aside.
3. Coat a pan with cooking spray over medium heat.
4. Sprinkle sea salt and pepper on scallops, add to pan, and sauté for 2 to 3 minutes on each side.
5. Spoon the sauce over scallops and serve.

Baked Lemon Chicken

3 pounds chicken breast

2 tablespoons extra-virgin olive oil

2 tablespoons chopped basil

¼ cup fresh lemon juice

1. Combine chicken, basil, lemon juice, and olive oil in a large bowl and toss together.
2. Refrigerate and let marinate for 2 hours.
3. Bake at 425°F for 50 to 60 minutes and serve.

Mushroom Steak

4 5-ounce top loin steaks, all visible fat trimmed

1 pound of mushrooms cleaned, trimmed, and cut into ¼-inch slices

1 tablespoon olive oil

½ cup low-sodium beef broth

1 teaspoon low-sodium soy sauce

½ teaspoon sea salt

½ teaspoon black pepper

4 cloves garlic

1 tablespoon chopped fresh thyme

1. In a large nonstick skillet, heat oil on medium-high.
2. Season both sides of steaks with sea salt and pepper.
3. Add steaks to skillet and cook until done to taste (3 to 5 minutes per side). Let sit for 5 minutes.
4. Meanwhile, place same skillet on medium heat. Add garlic and cook, stirring, for 30 seconds.
5. Add mushrooms and thyme; cook, stirring occasionally, until mushrooms are tender, about 3 to 5 minutes.

6. Add broth and soy sauce, deglazing pan by scraping browned bits from bottom of skillet with a spoon or spatula.

7. Cook, stirring occasionally, until liquid is reduced to a thin layer, 1 to 2 minutes.

8. Serve steaks with mushroom mixture over top, dividing evenly.

9. Garnish with additional thyme sprigs.

Seared Scallops with Vinaigrette Sauce

1 pound sea scallops

¼ cup soymilk

6 teaspoons olive oil, divided

2 cups fresh or frozen green peas

2 green onions, rinsed and thinly sliced

¼ teaspoon sea salt, divided in half

1 teaspoon fresh thyme leaves

1 teaspoon fresh lemon juice

2 teaspoons white wine vinegar

1 teaspoon minced fresh mint

½ teaspoon raw honey

1. Heat a skillet on medium-low and add 1 teaspoon oil and swirl to coat skillet.

2. Add green onions and ⅛ teaspoon salt and cook, stirring occasionally, until onions are softened and just starting to brown.

3. Add thyme, peas, and soymilk. Increase heat to medium and cook, stirring, until peas are heated through, about 5 minutes. Remove mixture from heat.

4. Scrape pea mixture into a blender and purée until smooth, adding a bit more milk to thin, if necessary.

5. Heat a large skillet on medium-high. Add 1 teaspoon oil and swirl to coat pan.

6. Add scallops, leaving a bit of space between each to prevent steaming. Sear scallops for about 3 minutes per side until golden brown and barely firm to the touch. Place scallops on a plate.

7. In a small bowl, whisk together remaining 4 teaspoons of oil, lemon juice, vinegar, 1 teaspoon water, mint, honey, and remaining sea salt.

8. To serve, spoon ? cup pea purée onto each of 4 plates and top with 4 scallops.

9. Spoon vinaigrette over top of scallops and serve.

Baked Halibut

2 5-ounce boneless, skin-on halibut fillets

1 teaspoon extra-virgin olive oil

1 large clove garlic, minced

2 teaspoons lemon zest

Juice from ½ lemon

1 tablespoon chopped parsley

Dash of sea salt

Dash of fresh ground black pepper

1. Preheat oven to 400°F.
2. In a large nonstick baking dish, add halibut, skin side down, and drizzle with oil.
3. Top with garlic, lemon zest, and 2 tablespoons of juice and parsley, dividing evenly; season with sea salt and pepper.
4. Bake for 12 to 15 minutes, until halibut flakes easily when tested with a fork.
5. Drizzle with remaining lemon juice and serve.

Collard Greens with Turkey Sausage

½ teaspoon chili powder

½ teaspoon paprika

¼ teaspoon sea salt

⅛ teaspoon each ground black pepper and
cayenne pepper

3 medium shallots, thinly sliced

1 tablespoon extra-virgin olive oil, divided

2 lean fresh turkey sausages with casings removed

1 pound of collard greens, stems removed
and leaves chopped

1. In a small bowl, mix together chili powder,
   paprika, salt, black pepper, and cayenne.
2. Heat 2 teaspoons oil in a large sauté pan on
   medium-high.
3. Add shallots and cook, stirring frequently, for
   3 minutes, until softened.
4. Heat remaining olive oil in pan. Add sausage
   and cook, breaking up meat with a wooden
   spoon, for about 3 minutes, until browned.
5. Stir remaining spice mixture and collard greens
   into pan. Cover and cook for 2 minutes.
6. Remove lid, stir, and cook for 2 more minutes.
7. Add shallot mixture back to pan, stir, and cook
   for 1 more minute, until heated through.

Glazed Salmon

4 salmon fillets

¼ cup tamari soy sauce

2 tablespoons raw honey

1 tablespoon rice vinegar

1 tablespoon ground ginger

¼ teaspoon cayenne pepper

⅛ teaspoon ground pepper

1. In a large bowl, combine the soy sauce, honey, vinegar, ginger, cayenne, and black pepper.
2. Add the salmon and marinate in a food storage bag for 2 hours.
3. Preheat the broiler and place salmon on a broiler rack for 8 to 10 minutes, until flaky with a fork. Serve.

Tuna Salad

3 cans water-packed tuna

½ cup nonfat Greek yogurt

2 teaspoons lemon juice

1 carrot, grated

1 hard-boiled egg

1 small tomato

½ small white onion, minced

½ teaspoon dried dill

1 teaspoon dried parsley

¼ teaspoon Dijon mustard

½ teaspoon garlic powder

1 teaspoon agave

Dash of sea salt

Black pepper to taste

> Mix all the ingredients together in one large bowl and serve.

Other Books by JJ Smith

If you'd like more information on products offered by JJ Smith, please see the website at www.JJSmithOnline.com.

The following books/ebooks can be found on the website:

- **Lose Weight Without Dieting or Working Out! (printed book/#1 bestseller)**

- **6 Ways to Lose Belly Fat Without Exercise (printed book)**

- **Who Else Wants to Look and Feel 10 Years Younger (DVD program)**

- **Why I Love Men: The Joys of Dating (printed book)**

- **Rich Diva: 10 Secrets of Six-Figure Women (ebook)**

- **101 Best Places to Meet Men (ebook)**

6 Ways to Lose Belly Fat Without Exercise!
www.JJSmithOnline.com

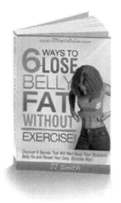

This book consists of six strategies for losing belly fat without exercise, and it includes over 50 belly fat recipes and a seven-day meal plan. If you'd like more information on this book or other products offered by JJ Smith, please visit:

www.JJSmithOnline.com

6 Ways to Lose Belly Fat Without Exercise! teaches the following:

✓ **Remove the FAT-Belly Foods and Add the 7 FLAT-Belly Foods**

✓ **5 Belly-Fat Blasting Supplements**

✓ **Clean the Gut, Lose the Gut: Learn the 2 Best Detox Methods That Help You Lose Belly Fat**

✓ **The #1 Hormonal Imbalance that Causes Belly Fat if You're Over 35!**

✓ **2 Surprising Habits That Cause Belly Fat**

✓ **A Little-Known Food Allergen That Causes Belly Fat and Bloating**

Lose Weight Without Dieting or Working Out!
www.JJSmithOnline.com

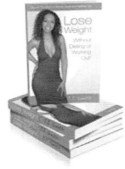

Want to lose weight without counting calories, starving yourself, giving up your favorite foods, or eating bland packaged foods? Would you like to look and feel younger and healthier than you have in years without diets and exercise? If you've answered yes to these questions, this book is for you! JJ Smith's revolutionary system teaches proven methods for permanent weight loss that anyone can follow, no matter their size, income level, or educational level. And the end result is a healthy, sexy, slim body.

You will learn how to....

- ✓ **Detoxify the body for fast weight loss**
- ✓ **Drop pounds and inches fast, without grueling workouts or starvation**
- ✓ **Lose up to 15 pounds in the first three weeks**
- ✓ **Shed unwanted fat by eating foods you love, including carbs**
- ✓ **Get rid of stubborn belly fat**
- ✓ **Trigger your 6 fat-burning hormones to lose weight effortlessly**
- ✓ **Eat foods that give you glowing, radiant skin**
- ✓ **Eat so you feel energetic and alive every day**
- ✓ **Get physically active without exercising**

This is your last stop on the way to a new fit and healthy you!
Look and feel younger than you have in years.
Create your best body—NOW

JJ Smith's Bio

www.JJSmithOnline.com

JJ Smith is the author of the #1 bestseller *Lose Weight Without Dieting or Working Out!* She is a nutritionist and certified weight-loss expert, and inspirational speaker. She has been featured on *The Steve Harvey Show*, *The Montel Williams Show*, *The Jamie Foxx Show*, and *The Michael Baisden Show*. JJ has made appearances on the NBC, FOX, CBS, and CW Network television stations, as well as in the pages of *Glamour*, *Essence*, *Heart and Soul*, and *Ladies Home Journal*. Since reclaiming her health, losing weight, and discovering a "second youth" in her forties, bestselling author JJ Smith has become the voice of inspiration to those who want to lose weight, be healthy, and get their sexy back! JJ Smith provides lifestyle solutions for losing weight, getting healthy, looking younger, and improving your love life!

JJ has dedicated her life to the field of healthy eating and living. JJ's passion is to educate others and share with them the natural remedies to stay slim, restore health, and look and feel younger. JJ has studied many philosophies of natural healing and learned from some of the great teachers of our time. After studying and applying knowledge about how to heal the body and lose weight, JJ went on to receive several certifications—one as a certified nutritionist and another as a certified weight-management expert. JJ received her certification as Nutritionist from the International Institute of Holistic Healing. JJ received her certification as a Weight-Management Specialist from the National Exercise and Sports Trainers Association

(NESTA). She is also a member of the American Nutrition Association (ANA).

JJ's current work, *Lose Weight Without Dieting or Working Out!*, is a revolutionary system that teaches proven methods for permanent weight loss that anyone can follow, no matter their size, income level, or educational level. And the end result is a healthy, sexy, slim body. JJ's breakthrough weight-loss solution can help you shed pounds fast by detoxifying the body, balancing your hormones, and speeding up your metabolism. You'll also learn which foods help you stay slim and which foods cause you to get fat. If you have been on a roller-coaster ride of weight loss, you will finally be able to get off that ride, lose weight, and stay slim for life!

JJ holds a B.A. in Mathematics from Hampton University in Virginia. She continued her education by completing The Wharton Business School Executive Management Certificate program. She currently serves as Vice President and Partner in an IT Consulting firm, Intact Technology, Inc., in Greenbelt, Maryland. JJ was also the youngest African American to receive a Vice President position at a Fortune 500 company. Her hobbies include reading, writing, and deejaying.

Made in the USA
San Bernardino, CA
22 April 2014